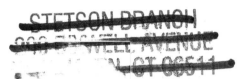

Pregnancy Information for Teens

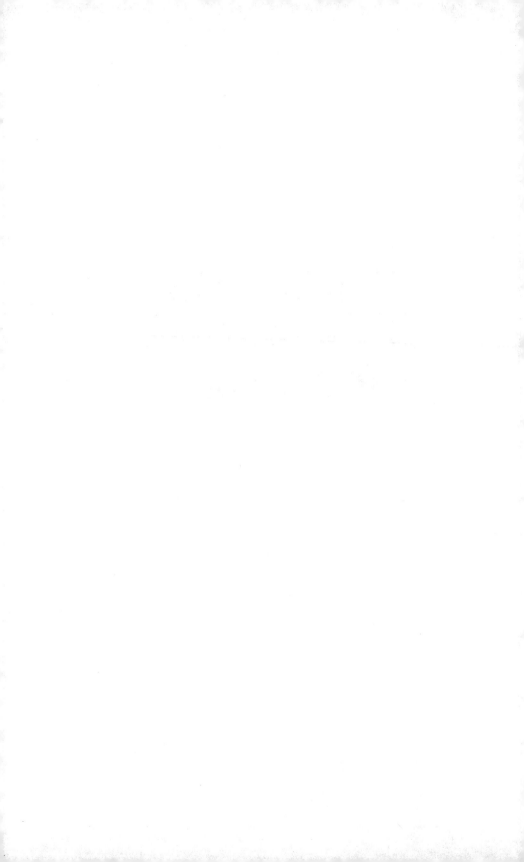

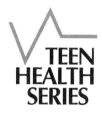

**TEEN
HEALTH
SERIES**

First Edition

Pregnancy Information for Teens

Health Tips About Teen Pregnancy And Teen Parenting

*Including Facts About Prenatal Care, Pregnancy
Complications, Labor And Delivery, Postpartum Care,
Pregnancy-Related Lifestyle Concerns, And More*

◆

Edited by Sandra Augustyn Lawton

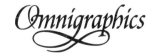

P.O. Box 31-1640 • Detroit, MI 48231-1640

Bibliographic Note

Because this page cannot legibly accommodate all the copyright notices, the Bibliographic Note portion of the Preface constitutes an extension of the copyright notice.

Edited by Sandra Augustyn Lawton

Teen Health Series

Karen Bellenir, *Managing Editor*
David A. Cooke, M.D., *Medical Consultant*
Elizabeth Collins, *Research and Permissions Coordinator*
Cherry Stockdale, *Permissions Assistant*
EdIndex, Services for Publishers, *Indexers*

* * *

Omnigraphics, Inc.

Matthew P. Barbour, *Senior Vice President*
Kay Gill, *Vice President—Directories*
Kevin Hayes, *Operations Manager*
David P. Bianco, *Marketing Director*

* * *

Peter E. Ruffner, *Publisher*
Frederick G. Ruffner, Jr., *Chairman*
Copyright © 2007 Omnigraphics, Inc.
ISBN 978-0-7808-0984-0

Library of Congress Cataloging-in-Publication Data

Pregnancy information for teens : health tips about teen pregnancy and teen parenting, including facts about prenatal care, pregnancy complications, labor and delivery, postpartum care, pregnancy-related lifestyle concerns, and more / edited by Sandra Augustyn Lawton.
   p. cm. -- (Teen health series)
   Summary: "Provides basic consumer information for teens about maintaining health during pregnancy, preparing for childbirth, and caring for a newborn. Includes index and resource information"--Provided by publisher.
   Includes bibliographical references and index.
   ISBN 978-0-7808-0984-0 (hardcover : alk. paper) 1. Teenage parents. 2. Teenage pregnancy. I. Lawton, Sandra Augustyn.
   HQ759.64.P72 2008
   618.200835--dc22
                                                                        2007016451

Table of Contents

Part Three: Staying Healthy During Your Pregnancy

Part Four: High-Risk Pregnancies And Pregnancy Complications

Part Five: Childbirth: Are You Prepared?

Part Six: Introducing Your Newborn

Part Seven: Teen Parenting Challenges

Part Eight: If You Need Help Or More Information

Preface

About This Book

According to the National Center for Health Statistics, 860,000 teens become pregnant each year, a situation that forces them to make life-changing decisions at an extremely emotional time. For the nearly half who choose to carry their pregnancies to term, prenatal care and birth options can seem bewildering. Furthermore, some pregnant teens may lack access to proper nutrition or may participate in risky activities, such as smoking, drinking alcohol, and taking drugs, which can have a negative effect on fetal health. Teen mothers face other problems as well. They must confront the difficult tasks of staying in school, earning an income, and finding a place to live.

Pregnancy Information For Teens discusses the choices to be made and the obstacles to be overcome when a young woman faces an unplanned pregnancy. It includes facts about abortion, adoption, prenatal care, nutrition, fetal development, and preparing for labor and delivery. For teens who choose to parent their infants, it offers information on how to care for a newborn, locate and pay for child care, and receive child support. It discusses the importance of completing an education and describes the public assistance programs that are available. An end section provides information about sources of help and directories of additional resources.

How To Use This Book

This book is divided into parts and chapters. Parts focus on broad areas of interest; chapters are devoted to single topics within a part.

Part One: Understanding The Problem Of Teen Pregnancy discusses the serious consequences teen pregnancy has on the mother, the child, and on society. It also presents information on two models for pregnancy prevention programs—abstinence-only and comprehensive sexuality education—and discusses differing viewpoints regarding the effectiveness of these approaches.

Part Two: If You Think You're Pregnant provides information on the signs and symptoms of pregnancy and the facts about pregnancy tests. After a pregnancy is confirmed, pregnant teens must make a difficult choice—abortion, adoption, or parenting. Individual chapters within this part discuss each of these alternatives.

Part Three: Staying Healthy During Your Pregnancy talks about what a pregnant teen must do—and not do—in order to have a healthy pregnancy. It includes information on prenatal care, tests and procedures, nutrition, and exercise. It also explains why alcohol, tobacco, illegal drugs, and some other substances must be avoided during pregnancy.

Part Four: High-Risk Pregnancies And Pregnancy Complications discusses various conditions that may be present before pregnancy that increase the risk of complications. These include asthma, diabetes, and eating disorders. It also discusses the kinds of prenatal concerns that warrant special care to prevent prematurity, birth-related injuries, or other adverse outcomes.

Part Five: Childbirth: Are You Prepared describes the many preparations that need to be made prior to childbirth, including birthing classes, birth plans, and choosing a birth location. It also presents information on the signs of labor, pain relief options, and facts about vaginal and cesarean delivery.

Part Six: Introducing Your Newborn gives teen mothers important information about what happens during a newborn's first few hours of life, including health assessments and screening tests. It also gives tips on taking care of a baby at home and answers questions about breastfeeding.

Part Seven: Teen Parenting Challenges discusses the many unique challenges adolescent parents face, including child care options, finding a place to live, and staying in school. Important facts are also presented relating to child custody and child support.

Part Eight: If You Need Help Or More Information describes public assistance that is available to teen parents, including supplemental nutrition and vaccine programs. It also discusses health insurance and how to get help paying for child care. The part concludes with directories of teen pregnancy resources, assistance resources for low-income pregnant women, and education resources for teen parents.

Bibliographic Note

This volume contains documents and excerpts from publications issued by the following government agencies: Administration for Children and Families (ACF); Centers for Disease Control and Prevention (CDC); Consumer Product Safety Commission (CPSC); Library of Congress; National Institute of Diabetes and Digestive and Kidney Diseases (NIDDK); National Women's Health Information Center (NWHIC); U.S. Department of Agriculture (USDA); U.S. Department of Education; U.S. Department of Housing and Urban Development (HUD); and the U.S. Food and Drug Administration (FDA).

In addition, this volume contains copyrighted documents and articles produced by the following organizations and individuals: A.D.A.M., Inc.; About, Inc.; Advocates for Youth; American College of Nurse-Midwives; American Pregnancy Association; Childbirth Connection; Mike Hardcastle; Juvenile Law Center; March of Dimes Birth Defects Foundation; Merck and Co., Inc.; National Association of Child Care Resource and Referral Agencies; National Campaign to Prevent Teen Pregnancy; National Eating Disorders Association; National Jewish Medical and Research Center; National Safety Council; Nemours Foundation; Northwest Community Healthcare; Parenting SA, Government of South Australia; Planned Parenthood Federation of America, Inc.; University of Michigan Health System; University of North Carolina at Chapel Hill; and Wiley Publishing, Inc.

Full citation information is provided on the first page of each chapter. Every effort has been made to secure all necessary rights to reprint the copyrighted material. If any omissions have been made, please contact Omnigraphics to make corrections for future editions.

The photograph on the front cover is from Problem Teens/BananaStock.

Acknowledgements

In addition to the organizations listed above, special thanks are due to the *Teen Health Series* research and permissions coordinator, Elizabeth Collins, and to its managing editor, Karen Bellenir.

About the *Teen Health Series*

At the request of librarians serving today's young adults, the *Teen Health Series* was developed as a specially focused set of volumes within Omnigraphics' *Health Reference Series*. Each volume deals comprehensively with a topic selected according to the needs and interests of people in middle school and high school.

Teens seeking preventive guidance, information about disease warning signs, medical statistics, and risk factors for health problems will find answers to their questions in the *Teen Health Series*. The *Series*, however, is not intended to serve as a tool for diagnosing illness, in prescribing treatments, or as a substitute for the physician/patient relationship. All people concerned about medical symptoms or the possibility of disease are encouraged to seek professional care from an appropriate health care provider.

If there is a topic you would like to see addressed in a future volume of the *Teen Health Series*, please write to:

Editor
Teen Health Series
Omnigraphics, Inc.
615 Griswold Street
Detroit, MI 48226

A Note about Spelling and Style

Teen Health Series editors use *Stedman's Medical Dictionary* as an authority for questions related to the spelling of medical terms and the *Chicago Manual of Style* for questions related to grammatical structures, punctuation, and other editorial concerns. Consistent adherence is not always possible, however, because the individual volumes within the *Series* include many documents from a wide variety of different producers and copyright holders, and the editor's primary goal is to present material from each source as accurately as is possible following the terms specified by each document's producer. This sometimes means that information in different chapters or sections may follow other guidelines and alternate spelling authorities. For example, occasionally a copyright holder may require that eponymous terms be shown in possessive forms (Crohn's disease *vs.* Crohn disease) or that British spelling norms be retained (leukaemia *vs.* leukemia).

Locating Information within the *Teen Health Series*

The *Teen Health Series* contains a wealth of information about a wide variety of medical topics. As the *Series* continues to grow in size and scope, locating the precise information needed by a specific student may become more challenging. To address this concern, information about books within the *Teen Health Series* is included in *A Contents Guide to the Health Reference Series*. The *Contents Guide* presents an extensive list of more than 13,000 diseases, treatments, and other topics of general interest compiled from the Tables of Contents and major index headings from the books of the *Teen Health Series* and *Health Reference Series*. To access *A Contents Guide to the Health Reference Series*, visit www.healthreferenceseries.com.

Our Advisory Board

We would like to thank the following advisory board members for providing guidance to the development of this *Series*:

Dr. Lynda Baker,
Associate Professor of Library and Information Science,
Wayne State University, Detroit, MI

Nancy Bulgarelli,
William Beaumont Hospital Library, Royal Oak, MI

Karen Imarisio,
Bloomfield Township Public Library, Bloomfield Township, MI

Karen Morgan,
Mardigian Library, University of Michigan-Dearborn, Dearborn, MI

Rosemary Orlando,
St. Clair Shores Public Library, St. Clair Shores, MI

Medical Consultant

Medical consultation services are provided to the *Teen Health Series* editors by David A. Cooke, M.D. Dr. Cooke is a graduate of Brandeis University, and he received his M.D. degree from the University of Michigan. He completed residency training at the University of Wisconsin Hospital and Clinics. He is board-certified in internal medicine. Dr. Cooke currently works as part of the University of Michigan Health System and practices in Ann Arbor, MI. In his free time, he enjoys writing, science fiction, and spending time with his family.

Part One

Understanding The Problem
Of Teen Pregnancy

Chapter 1

Teen Pregnancy: So What?

Teen pregnancy has serious consequences for the teen mother, the child, and to society in general.

Despite hitting the lowest level in 30 years, teen pregnancy rates are still high. In fact, 31% of teenage girls get pregnant at least once before they reach age 20, resulting in almost 750,000 teen pregnancies a year. At this level, the United States has the highest rate of teen pregnancy in the fully industrialized world.

Teen Pregnancy Is Bad For The Mother

- **Future prospects for teenagers decline significantly if they have a baby.** Teen mothers are less likely to complete school and more likely to be single parents. Less than one-third of teens that begin their families before age 18 ever earn a high school diploma. Only 1.5% earn a college degree by the age of 30.

- **There are serious health risks for adolescents who have babies.** Common medical problems among adolescent mothers include poor weight gain, pregnancy-induced hypertension, anemia, sexually transmitted diseases (STDs), and cephalopelvic disproportion. Later in life, adolescent mothers tend to be at greater risk for obesity and hypertension than women who were not teenagers when they had their first child.

About This Chapter: Information in this chapter is from "Teen Pregnancy—So What?" © 2006 The National Campaign to Prevent Teen Pregnancy. Reprinted with permission. For additional information, visit http://www.teenpregnancy.org.

- **Teen pregnancy is closely linked to poverty and single parenthood.** A 1990 study showed that almost one-half of all teenage mothers and over three-quarters of unmarried teen mothers began receiving welfare within five years of the birth of their first child. The growth in single-parent families remains the single most important reason for increased poverty among children over the last twenty years, as documented in the 1998 Economic Report of the President. Out-of-wedlock child bearing (as opposed to divorce) is currently the driving force behind the growth in the number of single parents, and half of first out-of-wedlock births are to teens. Therefore, reducing teen pregnancy and child bearing is an obvious place to anchor serious efforts to reduce poverty in future generations.

Teen Pregnancy Is Bad For The Child

- **Children born to teen mothers suffer from higher rates of low birth weight and related health problems.** The proportion of babies with low birth weights born to teens is 21 percent higher than the proportion for mothers age 20–24. Low birth weight raises the probabilities of infant death, blindness, deafness, chronic respiratory problems, mental retardation, mental illness, and cerebral palsy. In addition, low birth weight doubles the chances that a child will later be diagnosed as having dyslexia, hyperactivity, or another disability.

- **Children of teens often have insufficient health care.** Despite having more health problems than the children of older mothers, the children of teen mothers receive less medical care and treatment. In his or her first 14 years, the average child of a teen mother visits a physician and other medical providers an average of 3.8 times per year, compared with 4.3 times for a child of older child bearers. When they do visit medical providers, more of the expenses they incur are paid by others in society. One recent study suggested that the medical expenses paid by society would be reduced dramatically if teenage mothers were to wait until they were older to have their first child.

- **Children of teen mothers often receive inadequate parenting.** Children born to teen mothers are at higher risk of poor parenting because their mothers, and often their fathers as well, are typically too young to master the demanding job of being a parent. Still growing and developing themselves, teen mothers are often unable to provide the kind of environment that infants and very young children require for optimal development. Recent research, for example, has clarified the critical importance of sensitive parenting and early cognitive stimulation for adequate brain development. Given the importance of careful nurturing and stimulation in the first three years of life, the burden born by babies with parents who are too young to be in this role is especially great.

- **Children with adolescent parents often fall victim to abuse and neglect.** A recent analysis found that there are 110 reported incidents of abuse and neglect per 1,000 families headed by a young teen mother. By contrast, in families where the mothers delay child bearing until their early twenties, the rate is less than half this level, or 51 incidents per 1,000 families. Similarly, rates of foster care placement are significantly higher for children whose mothers are under 18. In fact, over half of foster care placements of children with these young mothers could be averted by delaying child bearing, thereby saving taxpayers nearly $1 billion annually in foster care costs alone.

- **Children of teenagers often suffer from poor school performance.** Children of teens are 50 percent more likely to repeat a grade; they perform much worse on standardized tests; and ultimately they are less likely to complete high school than if their mothers had delayed child bearing.

Teen Pregnancy Is Bad For Us All

- **The U.S. still leads the fully industrialized world in teen pregnancy and birth rates by a wide margin.** In fact, the U.S. rates are nearly double Great Britain's, at least four times those of France and Germany, and more than ten times that of Japan.

- **Teen pregnancy costs society billions of dollars a year.** There are nearly half a million children born to teen mothers each year. Most of these mothers are unmarried, and many will end up poor and on welfare. Each year the federal government alone spends about $9 billion to help families that began with a teenage birth.

• **Teen pregnancy hurts the business community's "bottom line."** Too many children start school unprepared to learn, and teachers are overwhelmed trying to deal with problems that start in the home. Forty-five percent of first births in the United States are to women who are either unmarried, teenagers, or lacking a high school degree, which means that too many children—tomorrow's workers—are born into families that are not prepared to help them succeed. In addition, teen mothers often do not finish high school themselves. It is not easy for a teen to learn work skills and be a dependable employee while caring for children.

• **A new crop of kids becomes teenagers each year.** This means that prevention efforts must be constantly renewed and reinvented. Between 1995 and 2010, the number of girls aged 15–19 is projected to increase by 2.2 million.

✔ Quick Tip

1. Thinking "it won't happen to me" is stupid; if you do not protect yourself, it probably will. Sex is serious. Make a plan.

2. Just because you think "everyone is doing it," does not mean they are. Some are, some aren't—and some are lying.

3. There are a lot of good reasons to say "no, not yet." Protecting your feelings is one of them.

4. You are in charge of your own life. Do not let anyone pressure you into having sex.

5. You can always say "no" even if you have said "yes" before.

6. Carrying a condom is just being smart; it does not mean you are pushy or easy.

7. If you think birth control "ruins the mood," consider what a pregnancy test will do to it.

8. If you are drunk or high, you cannot make good decisions about sex. Do not do something you might not remember or might really regret.

9. Sex will not make him yours, and a baby will not make him stay.

10. Not ready to be someone's father? It's simple: Use protection every time or do not have sex.

Source: Excerpted from "Thinking About The Right-Now: What Teens Want Other Teens To Know About Preventing Teen Pregnancy," © 2006 The National Campaign to Prevent Teen Pregnancy. Reprinted with permission. For additional information, visit http://www.teenpregnancy.org.

Chapter 2

A Statistical Look At Teen Pregnancy

Teenage Pregnancy

Teenage birth rates in this country have declined steadily since 1991. While this is good news, teen birth rates in the U.S. remain high, exceeding those in most developed countries. High teen birth rates are an important concern because teen mothers and their babies face increased risks to their health, and their opportunities to build a future are diminished.

- About 11 percent of all U.S. births in 2002 were to teens (ages 15 to 19). The majority of teenage births (about 67 percent) are to girls ages 18 and 19.

- About 860,000 teenagers become pregnant each year, and about 425,000 give birth.

- About one in three teenagers becomes pregnant before age 20.

- The teenage birth rate is declining. Between 1991 and 2002, the rate fell by 30 percent (from 61.8 per 1,000 women to 43). Still, in 2002 (the most recent year for which data are available), about 4 teenage girls in 100 had a baby.

About This Chapter: Information in this chapter is from "Teenage Pregnancy." © 2006 March of Dimes Birth Defects Foundation. All rights reserved. For additional information, contact the March of Dimes at their website www.marchofdimes.com.

• About 17 percent of teen mothers go on to have a second baby within three years after the birth of their first baby.

• Teen mothers are more likely than mothers over age 20 to give birth prematurely (before 37 completed weeks of pregnancy). In 2002, the 7,315 girls under age 15 who gave birth were more than twice as likely to deliver prematurely than women ages 30 to 34 (21 vs. 9 percent). Babies born too soon face an increased risk of newborn health problems and even death, as well as lasting disabilities.

♣ **It's A Fact!!**

In 2005, 34% of currently sexually active high school students did not use a condom during last sexual intercourse.

Source: Excerpted from "Sexual Risk Behaviors," June 2006, Centers for Disease Control and Prevention, Department of Health and Human Services.

Teen Mother's Health Affects Her Baby

• Teens too often have poor eating habits, neglect to take their vitamins, and may smoke, drink alcohol, and take drugs, increasing the risk that their babies will be born with health problems. Studies also show that teens are less likely than older women to be of adequate pre-pregnancy weight and/or to gain an adequate amount of weight during pregnancy (25 to 35 pounds is recommended for women of normal weight). Low weight gain increases the risk of having a low birth weight baby (less than 5½ pounds).

• Pregnant teens are more likely to smoke than pregnant women over age 25. In 2002, 13.4 percent of pregnant teens ages 15 to 17 and 18.2 percent of those ages 18 to 19 smoked, compared to 11.4 of all pregnant women. Smoking doubles a woman's risk of having a low birth weight baby and also increases the risk of pregnancy complications, premature birth, and stillbirth.

• Pregnant teens are least likely of all maternal age groups to get early and regular prenatal care. In 2002, 6.6 percent of mothers ages 15 to 19 years received late or no prenatal care (compared to 3.6 percent for all ages).

- A teenage mother is at greater risk than women over age 20 for pregnancy complications such as premature labor, anemia, and high blood pressure. These risks are even greater for teens that are under 15 years old. These youngest mothers also may be more than twice as likely to die of pregnancy complications than mothers ages 20 to 24.

- Three million teens are affected by sexually transmitted diseases annually out of a total of 12 million cases reported. These include chlamydia (which can cause sterility), syphilis (which can cause blindness, maternal death, and death of the infant), and HIV (the virus which causes AIDS, which may be fatal to the mother and infant).

Health Risks To The Baby

A baby born to a teenage mother is more at risk of certain serious problems than a baby born to an older mother.

- In 2002, 9.6 percent of mothers ages 15 to 19 years had a low birth weight baby (under 5.5 pounds), compared to 7.8 percent for mothers of all ages. The risk is higher for younger mothers: 11.3 percent of 15-year-old mothers had a low birth weight baby in 2002 (18,703 girls this age gave birth, and 2,112 had low birth weight babies) compared to 8.9 percent of women aged 19 (168,111 births, with 14,920 of low birth weight).

- Low birth weight babies may have organs that are not fully developed. This can lead to lung problems such as respiratory distress syndrome, bleeding in the brain, vision loss, and serious intestinal problems.

- Low birth weight babies are more than 20 times as likely to die in their first year of life as normal-weight babies.

Other Consequences Of Teenage Pregnancy

Life often is difficult for a teenage mother and her child.

- Teen mothers are more likely to drop out of high school than girls who delay childbearing. A 1997 study showed that only 41 percent of teenagers who have children before age 18 go on to graduate from high school compared to 61 percent of teens from similar social and economic backgrounds that did not give birth until ages 20 or 21.

- With her education cut short, a teenage mother may lack job skills, making it hard for her to find and keep a job. A teenage mother may become financially dependent on her family or on public assistance. Teen mothers are more likely to live in poverty than women who delay childbearing, and over 75 percent of all unmarried teen mothers go on welfare within 5 years of the birth of their first child.

- Teens may not have good parenting skills or have the social support systems to help them deal with the stress of raising an infant.

- A child born to an unmarried teenage high school dropout is 10 times as likely as other children to be living in poverty at ages 8 to 12.

- A child born to a teenage mother is 50 percent more likely to repeat a grade in school and is more likely to perform poorly on standardized tests and drop out before finishing high school.

Chapter 3

Questions And Answers About Pregnancy Among Sexually Experienced Teens

Pregnancy Among Sexually Experienced Teens

Despite impressive declines in teen pregnancy and childbearing since the early 1990s, a new analysis by the National Campaign to Prevent Teen Pregnancy underscores that the proportion of sexually experienced teens aged 15–19 (young people who have had sex at least once) who have gotten pregnant, or caused a pregnancy, remains startlingly high.

What's the top line from the analysis?

Almost one-third (31%) of all sexually experienced teen girls have been pregnant, and more than one in eight (13%) sexually experienced teen boys have caused a pregnancy. These rates are significantly higher among some groups of teens. For example, 52% of sexually experienced Hispanic teen girls and 40% of non-Hispanic black teen girls have been pregnant. Not surprisingly, the analysis

About This Chapter: Text under the heading "Pregnancy Among Sexually Experienced Teens" is from "Questions And Answers About Pregnancy Among Sexually Experienced Teens," © 2006 The National Campaign to Prevent Teen Pregnancy. Information under the headings "Teen Pregnancy Rates in the United States" and "Teen Birth Rates in the United States" is from "Teen Pregnancy Rates in the United States, 1972–2000" and "Teen Birth Rates in the United States, 1940–2004*," © 2005 The National Campaign to Prevent Teen Pregnancy. Reprinted with permission. For additional information, visit http://www.teenpregnancy.org.

also shows that teens who do not use contraception the first time they have sex, who have sex before age 15, or who have three or more sexual partners are much more likely to have been pregnant or caused a pregnancy.

What's new here? Hasn't the National Campaign said for some time that one-third of girls get pregnant by age 20?

Yes. However, the one-third formulation is based on pregnancy data from 2000 and is a longitudinal estimate of the proportion of teens that are likely to get pregnant before age 20. This new analysis provides a more recent (2002), point-in-time estimate of the proportion of teens that report they have been involved in a pregnancy. Moreover, this new analysis is based on data from the National Survey of Family Growth (NSFG), which permits examination of teen pregnancy rates by a number of variables, such as age at first sex and number of sexual partners, that would not be possible using vital statistics data.

♣ It's A Fact!!

- Teen girls who first have sex before age 15 are significantly more likely (46%) to have been pregnant than teens that first have sex at age 15 or older (25%). More than one in five teen boys (22%) who first have sex before age 15 have been involved in a pregnancy compared to 9% who first have sex at age 15 or older.

- More than one in three sexually experienced teen girls (37%) who have had three or more sexual partners have been pregnant compared to one in four sexually experienced girls (25%) who have had one or two sexual partners. Almost one in five sexually experienced teen boys (18%) who have had three or more sexual partners have been involved in a pregnancy compared to 9% of sexually experienced teen boys with two or fewer partners.

- Teens who used contraception the first time they had sex are less likely to report being involved in a pregnancy than those who did not.

Source: Excerpted from "One-Third of Sexually Experienced Teen Girls Have Been Pregnant," © 2006 The National Campaign to Prevent Teen Pregnancy. Reprinted with permission. For additional information, visit http://www.teen pregnancy.org.

What does the National Campaign hope to accomplish with this analysis?

Two things. First, letting teens know about the high risk of pregnancy among those who are sexually experienced might help motivate young people to make more cautious decisions about sex. That is, delay sex, have fewer sexual partners, or, for those who are sexually active, use contraception more consistently and carefully. Second, the impressive progress the nation has made in reducing teen pregnancy and births overall may have inadvertently convinced policy makers, and others who decide how resources are allocated, that preventing teen pregnancy is no longer a priority. This data makes clear that major efforts are still needed to help young people postpone pregnancy.

Why did the National Campaign decide to only look at sexually experienced teens?

In short, this analysis helps them better understand the actual consequences of teen sexual activity by highlighting data only for those teens known to be sexually experienced. Most analysis of teen pregnancy rates are based on data collected from all teens regardless of their sexual experience. This analysis, which is limited to those teens that have had sex, allows for a more focused analysis of the high proportion of pregnancy among sexually experienced teens.

Does this mean that previous pregnancy rates are unreliable?

Not at all. Most teen pregnancy rates reported in the press and elsewhere are based on data collected from teens regardless of sexual experience. This is important and useful information; for example, work in this area has made clear that recent declines in teen pregnancy and childbearing are due to more teens delaying sex and more consistent contraceptive use among those who are sexually experienced. The estimates presented in this analysis can be used as a guideline for determining the risk of pregnancy among sexually experienced teens. The National Campaign strongly suggests that individuals refer to the teen pregnancy rate published by either the National Center for Health Statistics (www.cdc.gov/nchs) or the Guttmacher Institute (www.guttmacher.org) for specific rates and numbers of teen pregnancies in the United States.

How reliable is this information?

This analysis may very well be a conservative estimate of how many teens actually do become pregnant or cause a pregnancy. Researchers have long noted that pregnancy is often underreported in surveys, especially among teens and for certain racial/ethnic, age, and gender population subgroups.

What data was used for this analysis?

The analysis is based on data collected in 2002 as part of the widely respected National Survey of Family Growth (NSFG), a periodic survey of fertility-related issues conducted by the Centers for Disease Control and Prevention, National Center for Health Statistics. The NSFG surveyed over 7,000 women and almost 5,000 men aged 15–44. More than 2,000 of the people surveyed are teens. The sample is designed to produce national, not state, estimates.

How was the data collected?

Interviews for the survey were administered in person, in home, by trained interviewers. Respondents were asked a number of questions including those detailed in this analysis as well as questions about sexually transmitted diseases, communication with parents, and sex education. For particularly sensitive questions, respondents were given a laptop computer and allowed to enter their own information anonymously.

Does this data suggest that the nation is failing to reduce adolescent pregnancy or childbearing?

Not at all. The teen pregnancy rate declined 28 percent between 1990 and 2000 (the most recent available data), and the teen birth rate declined by one-third between 1991 and 2004.

Teen Pregnancy Rates In The United States

The U.S. teen pregnancy rate for teens aged 15–19 decreased 28 percent between 1990 and 2000. After reaching 117 pregnancies per 1,000 females aged 15–19 in 2000. (Pregnancy data include births, abortions, and miscarriages.)

Figure 3.1 and Table 3.1 reflect pregnancies per 1,000 teen girls aged 15–19 in the United States and are the most recent national data available. Numbers have been rounded to the nearest whole number.

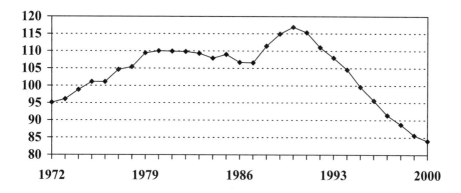

Figure 3.1. Teen Pregnancy Rates In The United States, 1972–2000

Table 3.1. Teen Pregnancy Rates in the United States, 1972–2000.

Year	Rate	Year	Rate	Year	Rate	Year	Rate
1972	95	1979	109	1986	107	1993	108
1973	96	1980	111	1987	107	1994	105
1974	99	1981	110	1988	111	1995	100
1975	101	1982	110	1989	115	1996	96
1976	101	1983	109	1990	117	1997	91
1977	105	1984	108	1991	115	1998	89
1978	105	1985	109	1992	111	1999	86
						2000	84

Henshaw, S.K. (2004). *U.S. teenage pregnancy statistics with comparative statistics for women aged 20–24.* New York: The Alan Guttmacher Institute.

Please note: There are three primary sources of U.S. pregnancy data on teens—those published by the National Center for Health Statistics (NCHS), United States Department of Health and Human Services (U.S. DHHS), those published by the National Center for Chronic Disease Prevention and Health Promotion (NCCDPHP), U.S. DHHS, and those published by the Alan Guttmacher Institute, a private, non-profit organization dedicated to protecting and expanding the reproductive choices of all women and men. For teen pregnancy statistics from NCHS and NCCDPHP, go to http://www.teenpregnancy.org.)

Teen Birth Rates In The United States

From 1940 to 1957, the teen birth rate increased 78 percent to a record high. The birth rate dropped fairly steadily from the end of the 1950s through the mid-1980s, but then increased 24 percent between 1986 and 1991. Between 1991 and 2004, the teen birth rate decreased 33.3 percent to a record low of 41.2 in 2004. Figure 3.2 and Table 3.2 reflect births per 1,000 teen girls aged 15–19 in the United States and are the most recent national data available.

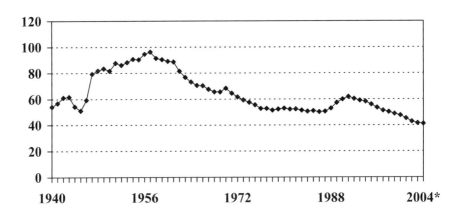

Figure 3.2. Teen Birth Rates In The United States, 1940–2004 (Birth rates for 2004 are preliminary.)

Table 3.2. Teen Birth Rates in the United States, 1940–2004*

Year	Rate	Year	Rate	Year	Rate	Year	Rate
1940	54.1	1956	94.6	1972	61.7	1988	53.0
1941	56.9	1957	96.3	1973	59.3	1989	57.3
1942	61.1	1958	91.4	1974	57.5	1990	59.9
1943	61.7	1957	90.4	1975	55.6	1991	61.8
1944	54.3	1960	89.1	1976	52.8	1992	60.3
1945	51.1	1961	88.6	1977	52.8	1993	59.0
1946	59.3	1962	81.4	1978	51.5	1994	58.2
1947	79.3	1963	76.7	1979	52.3	1995	56.0
1948	81.8	1964	73.1	1980	53.0	1996	53.5
1949	83.4	1965	70.5	1981	52.2	1997	51.3
1950	81.6	1966	70.3	1982	52.4	1998	50.3
1951	78.6	1967	67.5	1983	51.4	1999	48.8
1952	86.1	1968	65.6	1984	50.6	2000	47.7
1953	88.2	1969	65.5	1985	51.0	2001	45.3
1954	90.6	1970	68.6	1986	50.2	2002	42.9
1955	90.3	1971	64.5	1987	50.6	2003	41.6
						2004*	41.2

*Birth rates for 2004 are preliminary.

Sources: Ventura, S.J., Mathews, T.J., and Hamilton, B.E. (2001). Births to Teenagers in the United States, 1940–2000. *National Vital Statistics Reports, 49(10)*; Hamilton, B.E., Sutton, P.D., and Ventura, S.J. (2003). Revised Birth and Fertility Rates for the 1990s and New Rates for Hispanic Populations, 2000 and 2001: United States. *National Vital Statistics Reports 51(12)*; Martin, J.A., Hamilton, B.E., Sutton, P.D., Ventura, S.J., Menacker, F., and Munson, M.L., (2005). Births: Final Data for 2003. *National Vital Statistics Reports 54(2)*. Hamilton, B.E., Ventura, S.J., Martin, J.A., and Sutton, P.D. (2005). Preliminary Births for 2004. *Health E-Stats*. National Center for Health Statistics. Retrieved October 28, 2005 from http://www.cdc.gov/nchs/products/pubs/pubd/hestats/prelim_births/prelim_births04.htm.

Chapter 4

Pregnancy Prevention Programs:
No Consensus On Effectiveness

Adolescent Family Life And Abstinence Education Programs

Congress has provided funding for the prevention of teenage and out-of-wedlock pregnancies. This chapter discusses two programs that exclusively attempt to reduce teenage pregnancy.

The Adolescent Family Life Program

Adolescent Family Life (AFL): The program was enacted in 1981 as Title XX of the Public Health Service Act (P.L. 97-35). It is administered by the Office of Adolescent Pregnancy Programs, Department of Health and Human Services (HHS).

The AFL program was designed to promote family involvement in the delivery of services, adolescent premarital sexual abstinence, adoption as an alternative to

About This Chapter: Information under the heading "Adolescent Family Life And Abstinence Education Programs" is excerpted from "Reducing Teen Pregnancy: Adolescent Family Life and Abstinence Education Programs," by Carmen Solomon-Fears, Domestic Social Policy Division, CRS Report for Congress, Order Code RS20873, Updated October 4, 2004. Text under the heading "Sex Education Programs" is from "Sex Education Programs: Definitions and Point-by-Point Comparison," © 2004 Advocates for Youth. All rights reserved. Reprinted with permission.

early parenting, parenting and child development education, and comprehensive health, education, and social services geared to help the mother have a healthy baby and improve subsequent life prospects for both mother and child.

The AFL program authorizes grants for three types of demonstrations: (1) projects provide "care" services only (i.e., health, education, and social services to pregnant adolescents, adolescent parents, their infant, families, and male partners); (2) projects which provide "prevention" services only (i.e., services to promote abstinence from premarital sexual relations for pre-teens, teens, and their families); and (3) projects which provide a combination of care and prevention services.

Abstinence Education

1996 Welfare Reform: The 1996 welfare reform law stipulates that the term "abstinence education" means an educational or motivational program that (1) has as its exclusive purpose teaching the social, psychological, and health gains of abstaining from sexual activity; (2) teaches abstinence from sexual activity outside of marriage as the expected standard for all school-age children; (3) teaches that abstinence is the only certain way to avoid out-of-wedlock pregnancy, STDs, and associated health problems; (4) teaches that a mutually faithful monogamous relationship within marriage is the expected standard of human sexual activity; (5) teaches that sexual activity outside of marriage is likely to have harmful psychological and physical effects; (6) teaches that bearing children out-of-wedlock is likely to have harmful consequences for the child, the child's parents, and society; (7) teaches young people how to reject sexual advances and how alcohol and drug use increases vulnerability to sexual advances; and (8) teaches the importance of attaining self-sufficiency before engaging in sex.

Issues Regarding Adolescent Family Life And Abstinence Education Programs

Abstinence-Only Versus Comprehensive Sexuality Education: Advocates of the abstinence education approach argue that teenagers need to hear a single, unambiguous message that sex outside of marriage is wrong and harmful to their physical and emotional health. They argue that supporting both abstinence and birth control is hypocritical and undermines the strength of an abstinence-only message. They argue that abstinence clearly is the most

✤ **It's A Fact!!**

Although there is much research and many evaluations on both abstinence-only programs and comprehensive sexuality education programs, there is no consensus on the effectiveness of these approaches.

Source: CRS Report for Congress

effective means of preventing unwanted pregnancy and sexually transmitted diseases (including HIV/AIDS).

Advocates of the more comprehensive approach to sex education argue contend that such an approach allows young people to make informed decisions regarding abstinence, gives them the information they need to set relationship limits and to resist peer pressure, and also provides them with information on the use of contraceptives and the prevention of sexually transmitted diseases.

According to a 1997 report on research findings, at least four factors limit the conclusions that can be drawn from the many studies reviewed. First, the studies conducted to date are simply too few to evaluate each of the different approaches, let alone the various combinations of approaches. Second, many of these studies are limited by methodological problems or constraints. Third, these studies have often produced inconsistent results. And, fourth, there are very few replications of even the most promising programs that assess their impact in other types of communities and with other groups of youths.

Sex Education Programs

Definitions

Abstinence-Only Education teaches abstinence as the only morally correct option of sexual expression for teenagers. It usually censors information about contraception and condoms for the prevention of sexually transmitted diseases (STDs) and unintended pregnancy.

Abstinence-Only-Until-Marriage Education teaches abstinence as the only morally correct option of sexual expression for unmarried young people. Programs funded under the 1996 Welfare Reform Act must censor information about contraception and condoms for the prevention of STDs and unintended pregnancy.

Abstinence-Centered Education is another term normally used to mean abstinence-only education.

Comprehensive Sex Education teaches about abstinence as the best method for avoiding STDs and unintended pregnancy but also teaches about condoms and contraception to reduce the risk of unintended pregnancy and of infection with STDs, including HIV. It also teaches interpersonal and communication skills and helps young people explore their own values, goals, and options.

Abstinence-Based Education is another term normally used to mean comprehensive sexuality education.

Abstinence-Plus Education is another term normally used to mean comprehensive sexuality education.

Comparing Sex Education Programs

Comprehensive Sex Education

- teaches that sexuality is a natural, normal, healthy part of life

- teaches that abstinence from sexual intercourse is the most effective method of preventing unintended pregnancy and sexually transmitted diseases including HIV

- provides values-based education and offers students the opportunity to explore and define their individual values as well as the values of their families and communities

- includes a wide variety of sexuality related topics such as human development, relationships, interpersonal skills, sexual expression, sexual health, and society and culture

- includes accurate, factual information on abortion, masturbation, and sexual orientation

- provides positive messages about sexuality and sexual expression including the benefits of abstinence

- teaches that proper use of latex condoms, along with water-based lubricants, can greatly reduce, but not eliminate, the risk of unintended pregnancy and of infection with sexually transmitted diseases (STDs) including HIV

- teaches that consistent use of modern methods of contraception can greatly reduce a couple's risk for unintended pregnancy

- includes accurate medical information about STDs including HIV; teaches that individuals can avoid STDs

- teaches that religious values can play an important role in an individual's decisions about sexual expression; offers students the opportunity to explore their own and their family's religious values

- teaches that a woman faced with an unintended pregnancy has options: carrying the pregnancy to term and raising the baby, or carrying the pregnancy to term and placing the baby for adoption, or ending the pregnancy with an abortion

Abstinence-Only-Until-Marriage Education

- teaches that sexual expression outside of marriage will have harmful social, psychological, and physical consequences

- teaches that abstinence from sexual intercourse before marriage is the only acceptable behavior

- teaches only one set of values as morally correct for all students

- limits topics to abstinence-only-until-marriage and to the negative consequences of premarital sexual activity

- usually omits controversial topics such as abortion, masturbation, and sexual orientation

- often uses fear tactics to promote abstinence and to limit sexual expression

- discusses condoms only in terms of failure rates; often exaggerates condom failure rates

- provides no information on forms of contraception other than failure rates of condoms

- often includes inaccurate medical information and exaggerated statistics regarding STDs including HIV; suggests that STDs are an inevitable result of premarital sexual behavior

- often promotes specific religious values

- teaches that carrying the pregnancy to term and placing the baby for adoption is the only morally correct option for pregnant teens

Chapter 5

Questions And Answers About Birth Control And Emergency Contraception

Birth Control

What are the different birth control methods that I can use?

The following is a list of birth control methods with estimates of effectiveness, or how well they work in preventing pregnancy when used correctly, for each method:

- **Continuous Abstinence:** This means not having sexual intercourse (vaginal, anal, or oral intercourse) at any time. It is the only sure way to prevent pregnancy and protect against HIV and other STDs. This method is 100% effective at preventing pregnancy and STDs.

- **Periodic Abstinence or Fertility Awareness Methods:** Periodic abstinence means you do not have sex on the days that you may be fertile. These fertile days are approximately five days before ovulation, the day of ovulation, and one or more days after ovulation. Fertility awareness means that you can be abstinent or have sex but you use a barrier

About This Chapter: Information under the heading "Birth Control" is excerpted from "Birth Control Methods," July 2005. Text under the heading "Emergency Contraception" is excerpted from "Emergency Contraception," May 2006. The National Women's Health Information Center, U.S. Department of Health and Human Services, Office On Women's Health.

method of birth control to keep sperm from getting to the egg. These methods are 75 to 99% effective at preventing pregnancy.

- **The Male Condom:** Condoms are called barrier methods of birth control because they put up a block, or barrier, which keeps the sperm from reaching the egg. Only latex or polyurethane (because some people are allergic to latex) condoms are proven to help protect against STDs, including HIV. "Natural" or "lambskin" condoms made from animal products also are available, but lambskin condoms are not recommended for STD prevention because they have tiny pores that may allow for the passage of viruses like HIV, hepatitis B, and herpes. Male condoms are 84 to 98% effective at preventing pregnancy.

- **Oral Contraceptives:** They contain the hormones estrogen and progestin and are available in different hormone dosages. A pill is taken daily to block the release of eggs from the ovaries. They do not protect against STDs or HIV. The pill is 95 to 99.9% effective at preventing pregnancy.

- **The Mini-Pill:** Unlike the pill, the mini-pill only has one hormone, progestin, instead of both estrogen and progestin. Taken daily, the mini-pill thickens cervical mucus to prevent sperm from reaching the egg. It also prevents a fertilized egg from implanting in the uterus (womb). The mini-pill does not protect against STDs or HIV. Mini-pills are 92 to 99.9% effective at preventing pregnancy if used correctly.

- **Copper T IUD (Intrauterine Device):** An IUD is a small device that is shaped in the form of a "T." Your health care provider places it inside the uterus. The arms of the Copper T IUD contain some copper, which stops fertilization by preventing sperm from making their way up through the uterus into the fallopian tubes. If fertilization does occur, the IUD would prevent the fertilized egg from implanting in the lining of the uterus. The Copper T IUD can stay in your uterus for up to 12 years. It does not protect against STDs or HIV. This IUD is 99% effective at preventing pregnancy.

- **Progestasert® IUD (Intrauterine Device):** This IUD is a small plastic T-shaped device that is placed inside the uterus by a doctor. It contains the hormone progesterone. The progesterone causes the cervical mucus to thicken so sperm cannot reach the egg, and it changes the lining of the uterus so that a fertilized egg cannot successfully implant. The Progestasert® IUD can stay in your uterus for one year. This IUD is 98% effective at preventing pregnancy.

• **Intrauterine System or IUS (Mirena®):** The IUS is a small T-shaped device like the IUD and is placed inside the uterus by a doctor. Each day, it releases a small amount of a hormone that causes the cervical mucus to thicken so sperm cannot reach the egg. The IUS stays in your uterus for up to five years. It does not protect against STDs or HIV. The IUS is 99% effective.

• **The Female Condom:** Worn by the woman, this barrier method keeps sperm from getting into her body. It is made of polyurethane, is packaged with a lubricant, and may protect against STDs, including HIV. It can be inserted up to 24 hours prior to sexual intercourse. Female condoms are 79 to 95% effective at preventing pregnancy.

• **Depo-Provera®:** With this method, women get injections of the hormone progestin in the buttocks or arm every 3 months. It does not protect against STDs or HIV. It is 97% effective at preventing pregnancy.

• **Diaphragm, Cervical Cap, or Shield:** These are barrier methods of birth control. The diaphragm is shaped like a shallow latex cup. The cervical cap is a thimble-shaped latex cup. The cervical shield is a silicone cup that has a one-way valve that creates suction and helps it fit against the cervix. Before sexual intercourse, you use them with spermicide and place them up inside your vagina to cover your cervix (the opening to your womb). The diaphragm is 84 to 94% effective at preventing pregnancy. The cervical cap is 84 to 91% effective at preventing pregnancy for women who have not had a child and 68 to 74% for women who have had a child. The cervical shield is 85% effective at preventing pregnancy.

• **Contraceptive Sponge:** This is a barrier method of birth control. It is a soft, disk shaped device, with a loop for removal. It is made out of polyurethane foam and contains the spermicide nonoxynol-9. Before intercourse, you wet the sponge and place it, loop side down, up inside your vagina to cover the cervix. The sponge is 84 to 91% effective at preventing pregnancy in women who have not had a child and 68 to 80% for women who have had a child. The sponge is effective for more than one act of intercourse for up 24 hours. The sponge does not protect against STDs or HIV.

- **The Patch (Ortho Evra®):** This is a skin patch worn on the lower abdomen, buttocks, or upper body. It releases the hormones progestin and estrogen into the bloodstream. You put on a new patch once a week for three weeks, and then do not wear a patch during the fourth week in order to have a menstrual period. The patch is 98 to 99% effective at preventing pregnancy, but it appears to be less effective in women who weigh more than 198 pounds. It does not protect against STDs or HIV.

- **The Hormonal Vaginal Contraceptive Ring (NuvaRing®):** The NuvaRing® is a ring that releases the hormones progestin and estrogen. You squeeze the ring between your thumb and index finger and insert it into your vagina. You wear the ring for three weeks, take it out for the week that you have your period, and then put in a new ring. The ring is 98 to 99% effective at preventing pregnancy.

- **Surgical Sterilization (Tubal Ligation or Vasectomy):** These surgical methods are meant for people who want a permanent method of birth control. Tubal ligation or "tying tubes" is done on the woman to stop eggs from going down to her uterus where they can be fertilized. The man has a vasectomy to keep sperm from going to his penis, so his ejaculate never has any sperm in it. They are 99.9% effective at preventing pregnancy.

- **Non-surgical Sterilization (Essure® Permanent Birth Control System):** This is the first non-surgical method of sterilizing women. A thin tube is used to thread a tiny spring-like device through the vagina and uterus into each fallopian tube. Flexible coils temporarily anchor it inside the fallopian tube. A Dacron®-like mesh material embedded in the coils irritates the fallopian tubes' lining to cause scar tissue to grow and eventually permanently plug the tubes. It can take about three months for the scar tissue to grow, so it is important to use another form of birth control during this time. Then you will have to return to your doctor for a test to see if scar tissue has fully blocked your tubes. Essure® has been shown to be 99.8 % effective in preventing pregnancy.

Are there any foams or gels that I can use to keep from getting pregnant?

You can purchase what are called spermicides in drug stores. They work by killing sperm and come in several forms—foam, gel, cream, film, suppository, or tablet. They are inserted or placed in the vagina no more than one hour before intercourse. Spermicides are about 74% effective at preventing pregnancy.

How effective is withdrawal as a birth control method?

Withdrawal is not the most effective birth control method. Withdrawal is when a man takes his penis out of a woman's vagina (or pulls out) before he ejaculates, or has an orgasm. This stops the sperm from going to the egg. When a man's penis first becomes erect, there can be fluid called pre-ejaculate fluid on the tip of the penis that has sperm in it. This sperm can get a woman pregnant. Withdrawal also does not protect you from STDs or HIV.

Emergency Contraception

What is emergency contraception (or emergency birth control)?

Emergency contraception, or emergency birth control, is used to help keep a woman from getting pregnant after she has had unprotected sex (sex without using birth control).

Use emergency contraception if you did not use birth control; you were forced to have sex; the condom broke or came off; he did not pull out in time; you missed two or more birth control pills in a row; or you were late getting your shot.

♣ It's A Fact!!

If you are already pregnant, emergency contraception will not work.

Source: Excerpted from "Emergency Contraception," The National Women's Health Information Center.

♣ It's A Fact!!
How do I get emergency contraceptive pills (ECPs)?

Plan B (progestin-only) is sold over-the-counter to women who are 18 years of age or older. Women under the age of 18 will need a prescription. Women will have to show proof of age to buy Plan B. Plan B is sold at pharmacies or stores that have a licensed pharmacist on staff.

Source: Excerpted from "Emergency Contraception," The National Women's Health Information Center.

What are the types of emergency contraception?

There are two types—emergency contraceptive pills (ECPs) and intrauterine devices (IUDs).

There are two types of ECPs:

- **Plan B (progestin-only):** Made for use as emergency contraception. The two pills can be taken in two doses (one pill right away, and the next pill 12 hours later), or both pills can be taken at the same time.

- **Higher dose of regular birth control pills:** The number of pills in a dose is different for each pill brand, and not all brands can be used for emergency contraception. The pills are taken in two doses (one dose right away, and the next dose 12 hours later). Always use the same brand for both doses.

The other type of emergency contraception is the IUD. The IUD is a T-shaped, plastic device placed into the uterus (womb) by a doctor within five days after having sex. The IUD works by either keeping the sperm from meeting the egg or by keeping the egg from attaching to the uterus (womb). Your doctor can remove the IUD after your next period, or it can be left in place for up to ten years to use as your regular birth control.

Part Two

If You Think You're Pregnant

Chapter 6
Signs And Symptoms Of Pregnancy

Pregnancy symptoms differ from woman to woman and pregnancy to pregnancy; however, one of the most significant pregnancy symptoms is a delayed or missed menstrual cycle. Understanding pregnancy symptoms is important because each symptom may be related to something other than pregnancy. Some women experience pregnancy symptoms within a week of conception. For other women, symptoms may develop over a few weeks or may not be present at all. Below is a listing of some of the most common pregnancy symptoms.

Implantation Bleeding: Implantation bleeding can be one of the earliest pregnancy symptoms. About 6–12 days after conception, the embryo implants itself into the uterine wall. Some women will experience spotting as well as some cramping.

Other Explanations: Actual menstruation, altered menstruation, changes in birth control pill, infection, or abrasion from intercourse.

Delay/Difference in Menstruation: A delayed or missed menstruation is the most common pregnancy symptom leading a woman to test for pregnancy. When you become pregnant, your next period should be missed. Many women can bleed while they are pregnant, but typically the bleeding will be shorter or lighter than a normal period. This symptom is commonly explained by other reasons. If you have been sexually active and have missed a period, it is recommended that you take a test.

Other Explanations: Excessive weight gain/loss, fatigue, hormonal problems, tension, stress, ceasing to take the birth control pill, or breastfeeding.

Swollen/Tender Breasts: Swollen or tender breasts is a pregnancy symptom, which may begin as early as 1–2 weeks after conception. Women may notice changes in their breasts; they may be tender to the touch, sore, or swollen.

Other Explanations: Hormonal imbalance, birth control pills, or impending menstruation (PMS) can also cause your breasts to be swollen or tender.

Fatigue/Tiredness: Feeling fatigued or more tired is a pregnancy symptom, which can also start as early as the first week after conception.

Other Explanations: Stress, exhaustion, depression, common cold or flu, or other illnesses can also leave you feeling tired or fatigued.

Nausea/Morning Sickness: This well-known pregnancy symptom will often show up between 2–8 weeks after conception. Some women are fortunate to not deal with morning sickness at all, while others will feel nauseous throughout most of their pregnancy.

Other Explanations: Food poisoning, stress, or other stomach disorders can also cause you to feel queasy.

Backaches: Lower backaches may be a symptom that occurs early in pregnancy; however, it is common to experience a dull backache throughout an entire pregnancy.

Other Explanations: Impending menstruation, stress, other back problems, and physical or mental strains.

Headaches: The sudden rise of hormones in your body can cause you to have headaches early in pregnancy.

Other Explanations: Dehydration, caffeine withdrawal, impending menstruation, eyestrain, or other ailments can be the source of frequent or chronic headaches.

♣ It's A Fact!!

Can I Be Pregnant And Still Have Vaginal Bleeding?

Yes. Up to 25 percent of pregnant women have light vaginal bleeding, or spotting, during the first trimester. In most cases, spotting is not a sign of a problem. Light bleeding in the first trimester is often caused by the implantation of the fertilized egg in the wall of the uterus. This implantation bleeding usually happens 10 days or so after conception. Implantation bleeding is usually lighter and more irregular than a menstrual period.

But any vaginal bleeding during pregnancy or a suspected pregnancy should be taken seriously. If you are pregnant or think you are pregnant, you should always call your doctor if you have any bleeding. She will be able to figure out if it is a sign of a problem.

Sometimes bleeding in early pregnancy can signal trouble. Call the doctor immediately if you have the following:

• heavy bleeding

• bleeding with cramping, pain, fever, or chills

• bleeding that lasts more than 24 hours

Other common causes of vaginal bleeding in early pregnancy include the following:

• **Changes in the cervix:** During pregnancy, there is more blood flowing to the cervix, so it is more likely to bleed. Sexual intercourse during pregnancy can sometimes cause a small amount of vaginal bleeding. Also, many women have spotting after a pelvic exam.

• **Miscarriage:** Vaginal bleeding in the first trimester is sometimes a sign of a miscarriage.

• **Ectopic pregnancy:** Vaginal bleeding that often occurs along with some abdominal pain can be the sign of an ectopic pregnancy. An ectopic pregnancy occurs when the fertilized egg implants outside of the uterus, often in the fallopian tube. This is a serious condition that needs immediate attention. Ectopic pregnancies cannot produce a healthy baby. Plus, untreated ectopic pregnancies can seriously harm or kill the mother.

Source: From "Healthy Pregnancy," National Women's Health Information Center, U.S. Department of Health and Human Services, Office On Women's Health, February 2006.

Frequent Urination: Around 6–8 weeks after conception, you may find yourself making a few extra trips to the bathroom.

Other Explanations: Urinary tract infection, diabetes, increasing liquid intake, or taking excessive diuretics.

Darkening of Areolas: If you are pregnant, the skin around your nipples may get darker.

Other Explanations: Hormonal imbalance unrelated to pregnancy or may be a leftover effect from a previous pregnancy.

Food Cravings: While you may not have a strong desire to eat pickles and ice cream, many women will feel cravings for certain foods when they are pregnant. This can last throughout your entire pregnancy.

Other Explanations: Poor diet, lack of a certain nutrient, stress, depression, or impending menstruation.

Chapter 7

Pregnancy Tests

How do pregnancy tests work?

Pregnancy tests look for a special hormone in the urine or blood that is only there when a woman is pregnant. This hormone, human chorionic gonadotropin (hCG), can also be called the pregnancy hormone.

The pregnancy hormone, hCG, is made in your body when a fertilized egg implants in the uterus. This usually happens about six days after conception, but studies show that the embryo does not implant until later in some women. The amount of hCG increases drastically with each passing day you are pregnant.

What is the difference between pregnancy tests that check urine and those that test blood? Which one is better?

There are two types of pregnancy tests. One tests the blood for the pregnancy hormone, hCG. The other checks the urine for this hormone. You can do a urine test at home with a home pregnancy test. You need to see a doctor to have blood tests.

About This Chapter: Information in this chapter is from The National Women's Health Information Center, U.S. Department of Health and Human Services, Office On Women's Health, March 2006.

These days, most women first use home pregnancy tests (HPT) to find out if they are pregnant. HPTs are inexpensive, private, and easy to use. Urine tests will be able to tell if you are pregnant about two weeks after ovulation. Some more sensitive urine tests claim that they can tell if you are pregnant as early as one day after a missed period.

If a HPT says you are pregnant, you should call your doctor right away. Your doctor can use a more sensitive test, along with a pelvic exam, to tell for sure if you are pregnant. Seeing your doctor early on in your pregnancy will help you and your baby stay healthy.

♣ It's A Fact!!

Many home pregnancy tests claim they can tell if you are pregnant on the day you expect your period, but a recent study shows that most do not give accurate results this early in pregnancy. Waiting one week after a missed period will usually give a more accurate answer.

Source: The National Women's Health Information Center

Doctors use two types of blood tests to check for pregnancy. Blood tests can pick up hCG earlier in a pregnancy than urine tests can. Blood tests can tell if you are pregnant about six to eight days after you ovulate (or release an egg from an ovary). A quantitative blood test (or the beta hCG test) measures the exact amount of hCG in your blood, so it can find even tiny amounts of hCG. This makes it very accurate. Qualitative hCG blood tests just check to see if the pregnancy hormone is present or not, so it gives a yes or no answer. The qualitative hCG blood test is about as accurate as a urine test.

How do you do a home pregnancy test?

There are many different types of home pregnancy tests, or HPTs. Most drugstores sell HPTs over the counter. They cost between $8 and $20 depending on the brand and how many tests come in the box.

Most popular HPTs work in a similar way. The majority tells the user to hold a stick in the urine stream. Others involve collecting urine in a cup and then dipping the stick into it. At least one brand tells the woman to collect urine in a cup and then put a few drops into a special container with a dropper. Testing the urine first thing in the morning may help boost accuracy.

Then the woman needs to wait a few minutes. Different brands instruct the woman to wait different amounts of time. Once the time has passed, the user should inspect the "result window." If a line or plus symbol appears, you are pregnant. It does not matter how faint the line is. A line, whether bold or faint, means the result is positive.

Most tests also have a "control indicator" in the result window. This line or symbol shows whether the test is working or not. If the control indicator does not appear, the test is not working properly. You should not rely on any results from a HPT that may be faulty.

Most brands tell users to repeat the test in a few days, no matter what the results. One negative result (especially soon after a missed period) does not always mean you are not pregnant. All HPTs come with written instructions. Most tests also have toll-free phone numbers to call in case of questions about use or results.

Which brand of pregnancy test is the most accurate?

In a 2004 study, researchers tested the accuracy of 18 HPTs sold in retail stores. They found that only one brand consistently detected the low levels of hCG usually present on the first day of the missed period. This was the First Response, Early Result Pregnancy Test. The other tests missed up to 85% of pregnancies on the first day of the missed period. Most tests accurately confirmed pregnancies one week after the missed period.

How soon after a missed period can I take a home pregnancy test and get accurate results?

Many home pregnancy tests (HPTs) claim to be 99% accurate on the day you miss your period, but research suggests that most HPTs do not consistently spot pregnancy that early. When they do, the results are often so faint that they are misunderstood. If you can wait one week after your missed period, most home pregnancy tests will give you an accurate answer. Ask your doctor for a more sensitive test if you need to know earlier.

When a home pregnancy test will give an accurate result depends on many things. These include the following:

- **How long it takes for the fertilized egg to implant in the uterus after ovulation:** Pregnancy tests look for the hormone human chorionic gonadotropin (hCG) that is only produced once the fertilized egg has implanted in the uterine wall. In most cases, this happens about six days after conception; but studies show that in up to ten percent of women, the embryo does not implant until much later, after the first day of the missed period. Home pregnancy tests will

---

✔ Quick Tip
Calculating Your Dates:
Gestation, Conception, And Due Date

Gestational age, or the age of the baby, is calculated from the first day of the mother's last menstrual period. Since the exact date of conception is almost never known, the first day of the last menstrual period is used to measure how old the baby is.

Calculating Gestational Age

Last Menstrual Period: If the mother has a regular period and knows the first day of her last menstrual period, gestational age can be calculated from this date. Gestational age is calculated from the first day of the mother's last menstrual period and not from the date of conception.

Ultrasound: The baby can be measured as early as five or six weeks after the mother's last menstrual period. Measuring the baby using ultrasound is most accurate in early pregnancy. It becomes less accurate later in pregnancy. The best time to estimate gestational age using ultrasound is between the 8th and 18th weeks of pregnancy. The most accurate way to determine gestational age is using the first day of the woman's last menstrual period and confirming this gestational age with the measurement from an ultrasound exam.

Calculating Conception Date

In a Typical Pregnancy: For a woman with a regular period, conception typically occurs about two weeks after the first day of the last period. Most

be accurate as soon as one day after a missed period for some women but not for others.

- **How you use them:** Be sure to follow the directions and check the expiration date.

- **When you use them:** The amount of hCG in a pregnant woman's urine increases with time. The earlier after a missed period you take a HPT, the harder it is to spot the hCG. If you wait one week after a missed period to test, you are more apt to have an accurate result. Also, testing your urine first thing in the morning may boost the accuracy.

women do not know the exact date of conception, and their conception date is merely an estimate based on the first day of their last period.

Special Cases: Women who undergo special procedures, such as artificial insemination or in vitro fertilization, typically know the exact date of conception.

Calculating Due Date

Estimated Due Date: Based on the last menstrual period, the estimated due date is 40 weeks from the first day of the period. This is just an estimate since only about 5% of babies are born on their estimated due date.

Difficulties In Determining Gestational Age

Last Menstrual Period: For women who have irregular menstrual periods or women who cannot remember the first day of their last menstrual period, it can be difficult to determine gestational age using this method. In these cases, an ultrasound exam is often required to determine gestational age.

Baby's Growth: It is difficult to determine the gestational age in some cases because the baby is unusually large or small. Also, in some cases the size of the uterus in early pregnancy or the height of the uterus in later pregnancy does not match the first day of the last menstrual period. In these cases as well, it is difficult to obtain an accurate gestational age.

Source: Reprinted with permission from the American Pregnancy Association, http://www.americanpregnancy.org, © 2003. All rights reserved.

- **Who uses them:** The amount of hCG in the urine at different points in early pregnancy is different for every woman. Some women will have accurate results on the day of the missed period while others will need to wait longer.

- **The brand of test:** Some home pregnancy tests are more sensitive than others; therefore, some tests are better than others at spotting hCG early on.

I got a negative result on a home pregnancy test. Might I still be pregnant?

Yes. Most HPTs suggest women take the test again in a few days or a week.

Every woman ovulates at different times in her menstrual cycle, and embryos implant in the uterus at different times; therefore, the accuracy of HPT results varies from woman to woman. Other things can also affect the accuracy.

Sometimes women get false negative results (when the test says you are not pregnant and you are) when they test too early in the pregnancy. Other times, problems with the pregnancy can affect the amount of hCG in the urine.

If your HPT is negative, test yourself again in a few days or one week. If you keep getting a negative result but think you are pregnant, talk with your doctor right away.

Can anything interfere with home pregnancy test results?

Most medicines, over-the-counter and prescription, including birth control pills and antibiotics, should not affect the results of a home pregnancy test. Only medicines that have the pregnancy hormone hCG in them can give a false positive test result. A false positive is when a test says you are pregnant when you are not.

Sometimes medicines containing hCG are used to treat infertility (not being able to get pregnant). Alcohol and illegal drugs do not affect HPT results, but women who may become pregnant should not use these substances.

Chapter 8

Considering Abortion

Choosing Abortion

The chances are high that a woman will have more than one unplanned pregnancy in the course of her lifetime. More than one-third of all U.S. women will have an abortion by the time they are 45 years old. About six million women in the U.S. become pregnant every year. Half of those pregnancies are unintended.

The most common reasons a woman chooses abortion are as follows:

- She is not ready to become a parent.

- She cannot afford a baby.

- She doesn't want to be a single parent.

- She doesn't want anyone to know she has had sex or is pregnant.

- She is too young or too immature to have a child.

- She has all the children she wants.

- Her husband, partner, or parent wants her to have an abortion.

About This Chapter: Information in this chapter is from "Choosing Abortion" and "Procedures." Both are reprinted with permission from Planned Parenthood® Federation of America, Inc. © 2007 PPFA. All rights reserved. For additional information, visit www.plannedparenthood.org.

- She or the fetus has a health problem.

- She was a survivor of rape or incest.

Deciding If Abortion Is Right For You

Most women look to their husbands, partners, families, health care providers, clergy, or someone else they trust for support as they make their decision about an unintended pregnancy. And many women go to the clinic with their partner. But you don't have to tell anybody. Specially trained educators at women's health clinics can talk with you in private. You may bring someone with you. You will discuss your options—adoption, parenting, and abortion. You may be asked if someone is pressuring you to have an abortion.

Telling a parent is only required in states with mandatory parental involvement laws. Such laws force a woman under 18 to tell a parent or get parental permission before having an abortion. In most of these states, if she can't talk with her parents, or chooses not to, she can appear before a judge. The judge will consider whether she's mature enough to decide on her own. If not, the judge will decide whether an abortion is in the teen's best interests. In any case, if there are complications during the procedure, parents of minors may be notified.

Here are some things to consider if you are thinking about abortion. Answer true or false to the following statements:

1. No one is pressuring me to choose abortion.

2. I have strong religious beliefs against abortion.

3. I look down on women who have abortions.

4. I'd rather have a child at another time.

5. I can afford to have a child.

6. I can afford to have an abortion.

7. I care about what other people will think.

8. I can handle the abortion experience.

9. I'll go before a judge if necessary.

10. I would do anything to end this pregnancy.

Think about whether or not your answers suggest that abortion might be right for you.

> **☞ Remember!!**
>
> Teens are encouraged to involve parents in their decision to have an abortion, and most do have a parent involved.
>
> Source: Excerpted from "Choosing Abortion," Planned Parenthood® Federation of America, Inc.

Abortion Options

Early in pregnancy, you have two options for ending a pregnancy—medication abortion or abortion by vacuum aspiration. Medication abortion is the use of medicine to end a pregnancy. Vacuum aspiration is the use of gentle suction to end pregnancy.

Pregnancy is usually dated from the first day of the last menstrual cycle. You may choose medication abortion if you are early enough in pregnancy. This may be defined as up to 49, 56, or 63 days depending on how the medicine is taken. After 63 days, vacuum aspiration is your only abortion option during the first trimester, which is calculated as the first 14 weeks after the first day of a woman's last menstrual period.

After the first trimester, dilation and evacuation (D&E) is the most common abortion procedure. In a D&E, the cervix is slowly stretched open. The procedure is completed by emptying the uterus using a combination of suction and medical instruments. Another option, induction—in which premature labor is induced with various medicines—is not widely available.

Abortion Contraindications

Medication Abortion: You should not have medication abortion in the following situations:

• are too far along in pregnancy

- are unsure about having the procedure

- are unwilling to have a vacuum aspiration if needed

- cannot return for follow-up visits

- do not have access to a telephone, transportation, and back-up medical care

- have a known or suspected molar pregnancy—one in which the placenta develops abnormally

- have severe adrenal gland, heart, kidney, or liver problems

- take any medicine that should not be combined with the medications used in medication abortion—methotrexate, mifepristone, or misoprostol

- take anti-clotting medication or have blood-clotting disorders

- are unwilling to have your IUD—if you have one—removed before taking the medicine

Special considerations may be necessary if you are breastfeeding, have chronic heart, liver, respiratory, or kidney disease, have an infection or are sick, have severe anemia, have uncontrolled high blood pressure, or have any other serious health problems.

Vacuum Aspiration And D&E: You should not have vacuum aspiration or D&E if you are unsure about having the procedure.

Special considerations may be necessary if you are extremely overweight, are running a fever, have an infection in your uterus, have certain kinds of sexually transmitted infections, have certain serious health problems, have problems with anesthesia, or have seizures more than once a week.

Effectiveness

Medication Abortion: There are two types of medication abortion offered in the U.S.—mifepristone medication abortion and methotrexate medication abortion. Mifepristone and methotrexate affect the body differently. Mifepristone is used more often than methotrexate because it is more effective and more predictable. Mifepristone is 96–97 percent effective. Methotrexate is about 92–96 percent effective.

Some of the medicines used in medication abortion may cause serious birth defects if pregnancy continues. So, if they don't work, vacuum aspiration should be done.

Vacuum Aspiration And D&E: Vacuum aspiration and D&E abortion are more than 99 percent effective. Failure to end a pregnancy can happen due to unusual conditions: there can be more than one chamber in the uterus or the pregnancy may not be in the uterus. Repeated aspiration or other treatment may be needed if the initial procedure does not end the pregnancy.

Comparing Risks

If you choose abortion, you will also want to compare the benefits, risks, and side effects of each of your options. For example, both medication abortion and early vacuum aspiration are extremely safe, but current data suggest that medication abortion may carry a higher risk of death than early vacuum aspiration abortion. Even so, both procedures are much safer than abortion later in pregnancy or carrying a pregnancy to term.

Some women prefer medication abortion because they feel its benefits outweigh its risks. Other women prefer vacuum aspiration abortion because they feel its benefits outweigh its risks. Your clinician can help you decide, but the choice is up to you.

Procedures

When Abortions Are Performed

Most abortions in the United States—nearly 90 percent—are provided in the first trimester. Fewer than 10 percent take place in the second trimester, but after 24 weeks of pregnancy, abortions are performed only for serious health reasons. Less than one-tenth of one percent of abortions happen during this time.

Preparing For An Abortion

You will need to discuss your options, sign a consent form, give a medical history, have laboratory tests, and have a physical exam—often including an ultrasound.

♣ It's A Fact!!
The Earlier, The Better

Try to arrange an abortion procedure as soon as you have made up your mind to have one. Earlier abortions are easier and safer than abortions later in pregnancy. They may also cost less.

Source: Excerpted from "Procedures," Planned Parenthood® Federation of America, Inc.

How Medication Abortion Works

There are three steps for medication abortion:

Step One: Your clinician will give you a dose of either mifepristone or methotrexate at the clinic. Mifepristone blocks the hormone progesterone. Without progesterone, the lining of the uterus breaks down, ending the pregnancy. Methotrexate stops the growth of the pregnancy in the uterus. It can also stop the growth of pregnancies that develop in a fallopian tube, which are called ectopic pregnancies.

Step Two: You will take a second medication called misoprostol. Misoprostol softens the cervix and causes the uterus to contract and empty.

You and your clinician will plan the timing and place for the second step; you may take the second medicine at home, or you may need to return to the clinic. Your clinician will give you instructions on how to take it.

You will take the misoprostol up to three days after taking mifepristone or about five days after taking methotrexate.

After you take the misoprostol, you will most likely start to bleed heavily within hours or days. This is the abortion. You may see large blood clots or tissue at the time of the abortion.

Step Three: You will return to your clinician for a follow-up visit within two weeks. Your clinician needs to make sure the abortion is complete and that you are well. You will need an ultrasound or blood test.

How Vacuum Aspiration And D&E Work

Vacuum aspiration empties the uterus with gentle suction of a hand-held suction device or with machine-operated suction. When it is performed with a manual suction device, it is sometimes called manual vacuum aspiration or MVA. When it is performed with machine-operated suction, it is sometimes called dilation and suction curettage or D&C.

During a vacuum aspiration abortion the following happens:

- Your uterus will be examined.

- A speculum will be inserted into your vagina.

- You may be offered sedation.

- The clinician may inject a numbing medication into or near your cervix.

- The opening of the cervix may be stretched with dilators, a series of increasingly thick rods, or you may have special absorbent dilators inserted that will absorb fluid and slowly stretch open your cervix. Sometimes absorbent dilators are inserted the night before and work as you sleep. Medication may also be used instead of, or along with, dilators to help open the cervix. You may also be given antibiotics to prevent infection.

- A tube is inserted through the cervix into the uterus.

- Either a hand-held suction device (MVA) or a suction machine (D&C) gently empties the uterus.

- A separate curette may be used to help remove the tissue that lines the uterus.

During a D&E abortion the following happens:

- Your uterus will be examined.

- A speculum will be inserted into your vagina.

- You may have special absorbent dilators inserted as early as the night before that will absorb fluid and slowly stretch open your cervix as you sleep. Medication may also be used instead of, or along with, dilators to help open the cervix. You may also be given antibiotics to prevent infection.

- You may be offered sedation or IV medication to make you more comfortable.

- A local numbing medication is injected into or near the cervix.

- The dilators are removed.

- The uterus is emptied with medical instruments and suction.

Make a follow-up appointment in two to four weeks after your vacuum aspiration or D&E abortion.

How Long An Abortion Takes

Medication Abortion: Medication abortion is a process that begins immediately after taking mifepristone or methotrexate. Some women may begin bleeding before taking misoprostol. For most, the bleeding and cramping begin after taking the misoprostol.

More than 50 percent of women who use mifepristone abort within four or five hours after taking misoprostol. Bleeding may continue for about 13 days. Spotting can last for a few weeks. About 92 percent of mifepristone abortions are completed within a week. About 75 percent of methotrexate abortions are completed within a week, but in 15–20 percent of women it can take up to four weeks.

Vacuum Aspiration And D&E: A vacuum aspiration procedure takes about 10 minutes. A D&E procedure usually takes between 10 and 20 minutes. Additional time is needed for client education, a physical exam, reading and signing forms, and a recovery period of about one hour.

What To Expect After An Abortion

Medication Abortion: You will be given written after-care instructions and a 24-hour emergency phone number to take home with you.

You should feel better each day after the abortion. You may have some bleeding for up to four weeks after. You may use pads or tampons, but using pads makes it easier to keep track of your bleeding.

You may want to stay home and relax on the day that you take the misoprostol or whenever your bleeding starts. You can usually return to work or other normal activities in the next day or two.

Until your follow-up visit, do not take aspirin. If you had methotrexate abortion, do not take vitamins with folic acid.

A low dose of misoprostol will be present in breast milk around the time of its use. It may cause an infant to have diarrhea. Talk with your clinician if you are breastfeeding.

Vacuum Aspiration And D&E: You will be given written after-care instructions and a 24-hour emergency phone number to take home with you.

You may have cramps. You may want to relax for the rest of the day. You may shower as soon as you wish. Do not take baths, douche, or use vaginal medications. Do not drive after the procedure if you've had sedation. You can usually return to work or other normal activities the next day. Recovery after D&E may take longer.

Some vaginal bleeding is normal after an abortion. It is normal to pass a few clots the size of a quarter. It is also normal to have no bleeding, spotting that lasts up to six weeks, heavy bleeding for a few days, or bleeding that stops and starts again. You may use pads or tampons, but using pads makes it easier to keep track of your bleeding.

✎ What's It Mean?

Dilation and Suction Curettage (D&C): When vacuum aspiration is performed with machine-operated suction.

Dilation and Evacuation (D&E): The most common abortion procedure. The cervix is slowly stretched open. The procedure is completed by emptying the uterus using a combination of suction and medical instruments.

Induction: Premature labor is induced with various medicines.

Medication Abortion: The use of medicine to end a pregnancy.

Vacuum Aspiration: The use of suction to end pregnancy.

Source: From "Choosing Abortion" and "Procedures," reprinted with permission from Planned Parenthood® Federation of America, Inc. © 2007 PPFA. All rights reserved. For additional information, visit www.plannedparenthood.org.

Warning Signs After An Abortion

Call your clinician right away if at any time you have any of the following:

- heavy bleeding—pass clots larger than a lemon or soak through more than two maxi pads an hour, for two hours or more in a row

- pain or discomfort not helped by medication, rest, a hot water bottle, or a heating pad

- a fever

- vomiting for more than four to six hours and are not able to keep anything down

- an unpleasant smelling vaginal discharge

- signs of a continuing pregnancy

During a medication abortion, feeling sick including abdominal pain or discomfort, diarrhea, nausea, vomiting, or weakness more than 24 hours after taking misoprostol could be a sign of serious infection. Contact your clinician right away if you have any of these symptoms. Do not wait for your follow-up appointment.

You may need another visit with your provider. Rarely, women need vacuum aspiration or hospitalization after medication abortion. Take your medication guide with you if you need to visit an emergency room, hospital, or clinician who did not give you the medicine.

Getting Your Period After An Abortion

Abortion begins a new menstrual cycle. You should have a regular period in four to eight weeks.

Having Sex After An Abortion

You can get pregnant very soon after an abortion. Discuss birth control options with your clinician.

Many clinicians recommend that you not have vaginal intercourse or insert anything except a tampon into your vagina for one week after the abortion.

Cost

Costs vary from community to community based on regional and local expenses.

Medication Abortion: Nationwide, cost ranges from $350 to $650. Cost may be more or less, depending on whatever additional tests, visits, or exams are needed.

Vacuum Aspiration And D&E: Costs vary depending on how long you've been pregnant and where you go. Nationwide, the cost ranges from about $350 to $700 for abortion in the first trimester. Hospitals generally cost more.

Where To Get An Abortion

Contact Planned Parenthood at 800-230-PLAN, other women's health care centers, or your private clinician. Planned Parenthood centers that do not provide abortion can refer you to someone who does. Or you can call the National Abortion Federation at 800-772-9100.

Chapter 9

Are You Pregnant And Thinking About Adoption?

If you are pregnant and not sure that you want to keep the baby, you might be thinking about adoption.

Pregnancy causes many changes, both physical and emotional. It can be a very confusing time for a woman, even in the best of circumstances. Talking to a counselor about your options might help, but how do you start?

Whom can I talk to about my options?

If you want to talk to a professional about your options, there are different places you can go. Counseling at the places listed below will be free or cost very little.

- **Crisis Pregnancy Center:** This is a place where they talk only to pregnant women. It might even have a maternity center attached where you could live until the baby is born.

- **Family Planning Clinic:** This is a place where women get birth control information or pregnancy tests.

About This Chapter: Information in this chapter is from Child Welfare Information Gateway, Administration for Children and Families, U.S. Department of Health and Human Services (www.childwelfare.gov), updated July 2006.

- **Adoption Agency:** This choice is good if you are already leaning strongly in the direction of adoption.

- **Health Department or Social Services:** A food stamps or welfare worker can tell you which clinic or department is the right one.

- **Mental Health Center or Family Service Agency:** Counselors at these places help all kinds of people in all kinds of situations.

A counselor may have strong feelings about adoption, abortion, and parenting a child. Nevertheless, those feelings should not influence their professional advice or the treatment provided to you. In order to make up your own mind, it is important for you to get clear answers from your counselor to the following three questions:

1. If I feel I cannot carry my pregnancy to term, how will you help me?

2. If I decide to take care of my baby myself, how will you help me do that?

3. If I want to place my baby for adoption, will you help me find an adoption agency or attorney who will listen to what I think is right for me?

If you are not happy with the answers you get, you may wish to find a counselor at another place. Child Welfare Information Gateway (http://www.childwelfare.gov) can tell you about crisis pregnancy centers and adoption agencies in each state and can also help you find other counseling agencies in your area.

Should I place my child for adoption?

The decision to place a child for adoption is a difficult one. It is an act of great courage and much love.

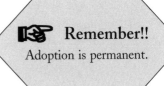

Remember!!
Adoption is permanent.

The adoptive parents will raise your child and have legal authority for his or her welfare. You need to think about the following questions as you make your decision:

- **Have I explored all possibilities?** Are you only thinking about adoption because you have money problems or because your living situation is difficult? These problems might be temporary. Have you called

Social Services to see what they can do or asked friends and family if they can help? If you have done these things and still want adoption, you will feel more content with your decision.

- **Will the adoptive parents take good care of my child?** Prospective adoptive parents are carefully screened and give a great deal of information about themselves. They are visited in their home several times by a social worker and must provide personal references. They are taught about the special nature of adoptive parenting before an adoption takes place. By the time an agency has approved adoptive parents for placement, they have gotten to know them very well and feel confident they would make good parents.

- **Will my child wonder why I placed him (or her) for adoption?** Probably. Most adopted adults realize that their birth parents placed them for adoption out of love and because it was the best they knew how to do. Hopefully your child will come to realize that a lot of his or her wonderful traits come from you, and if you have an open adoption, it is likely that you will be able to explain to the child why you chose adoption.

- **Why am I placing my child for adoption?** If your answer is because it is what you, or you and your partner think is best, then it is a good decision. Now it is time to move forward and not feel guilty.

What are the different types of adoption?

There are two types of adoptions, confidential and open.

Confidential: The birth parents and the adoptive parents never know each other. Adoptive parents are given background information about you and the birth father that they would need to help them take care of the child, such as medical information.

Open: The birth parents and the adoptive parents know something about each other. There are different levels of openness, such as the following:

- **Least Open:** You will read about several possible adoptive families and pick the one that sounds best for your baby. You will not know each other's names.

- **More Open:** You and the possible adoptive family will speak on the telephone and exchange first names.

- **Even More Open:** You can meet the possible adoptive family. Your social worker or attorney will arrange the meeting at the adoption agency or attorney's office.

- **Most Open:** You and the adoptive parents share your full names, addresses, and telephone numbers. You stay in contact with the family and your child over the years by visiting, calling, or writing each other. Fifteen states have enacted laws that recognize post-adoption contact between adoptive and birth families if the parties have voluntarily agreed to this plan.

How do I arrange an adoption through an agency?

In all states, you can work with a licensed child-placing (adoption) agency. In all but four states, you can also work directly with an adopting couple or their attorney without using an agency.

Private adoption agencies arrange most infant adoptions. To find private adoption agencies in your area, either contact Child Welfare Information Gateway or look in the yellow pages of your local phone book under "Adoption Agencies."

There are several types of private adoption agencies. Some are for profit and some are nonprofit. Some work with prospective adoptive parents of a particular religious group, though they work with birth parents of all religions.

When you contact adoption agencies, ask the social workers as many questions as you need to ask so that you understand the agencies' rules. Some questions you will want to ask are as follows:

- Will I get counseling all through my pregnancy, after I sign the papers allowing my child to be adopted, and after my baby is gone?

- Can my baby's father and other people who are important to me join me in counseling if they want to?

- What kind of financial help can I get? What kind of medical and legal help will I have? Can I get help with medical and legal expenses?

- What will I get to know about the people who adopt my baby? May I tell you what I think are important traits for parents to have? How do you know the adoptive parents are good people? May I meet them if I want or know their names? Will I ever be able to have contact with them or my child? Will I ever know how my child turns out?

- What information will you provide to the adoptive parents about my family and me?

The agency social worker will ask you questions to find out some information about you and the baby's father, such as your medical histories, age, race, physical characteristics, whether you have been to see a doctor since you became pregnant, whether you have been pregnant or given birth before, and whether you smoked cigarettes, took any drugs, or drank any alcohol since you became pregnant. The social worker asks these questions so that the baby can be placed with parents who will be fully able to care for and love the baby, not so that she can turn you down.

How do I arrange a private adoption?

An adoption arranged without an adoption agency is called an independent or private adoption. It is legal in all states except Connecticut, Delaware, Massachusetts, and Minnesota. With a private adoption, you need to find an attorney to represent you. Look for an attorney who will not charge you a fee if you decide not to place your baby for adoption. You also need to find adoptive parents.

To Find An Attorney

Legal Aid: This is a service available in most communities for people who cannot afford a private attorney. Sometimes it is located at a university law school. (Some states allow the adopting parents to pay your legal fee; so going to Legal Aid may not be necessary.)

State Attorney Association or the American Academy of Adoption Attorneys: These groups can refer you to an attorney who handles adoptions in your area. Contact Child Welfare Information Gateway for the address and telephone number of your state attorney association. You can contact the American Academy of Adoption Attorneys at P.O. Box 33053, Washington, DC 20033-0053.

To Find Adoptive Parents

Personal Ads: Some newspapers carry personal ads from people seeking to adopt. You call the number in the ad and get to know each other over the telephone. If you think you want to work with

✔ Quick Tip

When looking for adoptive parents, personal referrals are always good. Ask friends and family if they know any attorneys or possible adoptive parents.

the couple, have your attorney call their attorney. The attorneys will work out all the arrangements according to what you and the adoptive parents want and the laws of your state.

Your Doctor: He or she may know about couples that are seeking a child and be able to help arrange the adoption.

Adoptive Parent Support Groups: Parents who have already adopted may know other people seeking to adopt. You can find out more about these groups from Child Welfare Information Gateway.

National Matching Services: These services help birth parents and adoptive parents find one another. Contact Child Welfare Information Gateway for more information.

How do I arrange for future contact with my child if I want it?

If you decide on a confidential adoption, you may still wish to make sure that your child can contact you in the future. Many states, and some private national organizations, have set up adoption registries to help people find one another.

A registry works like this. You leave the information about the birth of the child and your address and telephone number. You must keep your address and telephone number current. You can register at any time, even years after the child is born.

When your child is an adult, he or she can call or write this registry. If what the child knows about his or her birth matches what the registry has, the registry will release your current address and telephone number to the child, and you could be contacted.

There is another way to ensure that your child can contact you if he or she wishes. Some adoption agencies and attorneys who arrange private adoptions will hold a letter in their file in which you say why you chose adoption and how to get in touch with you if the child ever wants to. If the agency or attorney that you are working with will not agree to do this, you may wish to work with somebody else.

Chapter 10

If You Choose To Raise Your Child

There are lots of good things about being a young parent, but there can also be extra stresses and problems. There are times when you might still feel you would like to have someone to take care of you. There will be other times when you want to be free to do what you like without the responsibility of a child.

It will make a difference if you are on your own with your child or if you have a partner. It will make a difference if you have the blessing and practical support of your family or feel unsupported by family and friends. These things can make it much easier or much harder to be a teenage parent. Being a parent is one of the most difficult things you can do; but it is one of the most important, and it can be fun.

Looking After Your Child

Children need love and affection. Give your child lots of cuddles, and tell him you love him many times a day.

Children are eager to learn and need lots of things to do. When they are very young, their parents are their best playmates. They like to be danced with, talked to, read to, sung to, and to be taken for walks. They like for you to lie on the floor and let them crawl over you and for you to play with them and their toys.

About This Chapter: Information in this chapter is from "Teenage Parents." Copyright © Parenting SA, Government of South Australia; information updated 2006.

Children need your time. They want you to be around them and to take notice of them. This might mean giving up things you want to do, and it might mean making out you are interested in what they are doing, even when you do not feel like it. Your time and attention helps your child to feel loved.

Young children need to be closely watched, especially near water (even diaper pails). Children can get into all sorts of things when you are busy. It is important to make your house and outdoor area as safe as possible. Soaps, laundry detergents, and medicines need to be kept in a high, locked cabinet.

The best toys for young children are often ones you do not need to buy. Children love saucepans and saucepan lids, pegs or lids to put into containers, walks in the park and picnics, homemade play dough, pitchers, and water to pour, cushions on the floor to crawl over, and cardboard boxes of different sizes to crawl through and into and to make into play houses.

Change the toys occasionally to give variety. Keep a special toy for a treat.

Join a library (and toy library) to borrow books and toys at no cost. Take him to a playground or join a play group.

Looking After Yourself

Children need you to look after them, but you cannot do this well if you do not look after yourself.

One of the things you may find hard as a young parent is the loss of your friends who do not have children. Sometimes you feel that you do not have anything to talk about anymore. By joining a young parents' group you will make new friends who have similar lives to yours. Here you can have fun, your children can play with other children, and you can talk over the same problems you share with other young parents.

It is okay to need your own space. Arrange for someone reliable to care of your child so you can have a night out, go shopping, or do something special. All parents need a break.

All parents have times when they get really busy and times when they get upset. Take a break, go outside, call a friend or someone you trust and talk about it. Always make sure your child is safe first. Often being outside can make you feel less stressed, so taking your baby for a walk around the block, or your toddler to the local playground, can help.

Even though you are a young parent, it is important to still plan for the future. Some areas have school programs designed for young parents and may have child care on site.

Getting Help

Most parents want to be seen as being able to cope well. They want others to think that they know how to be a good parent. Sometimes there is a fear that asking for advice means you are not a good parent, and this is quite wrong.

Young parents often believe they can do everything themselves and do not want older adults interfering. No matter how old parents are, they need information, support, and advice from others, and everyone needs to feel that it is safe to say we do not know sometimes without feeling ashamed.

Ask other young parents where they have found support. Sometimes young parents feel that they are being judged when they go to an agency, a doctor, or a clinic for help. It is important to look around until you find someone with whom you feel comfortable.

If you have problems with professionals not understanding what you want, think about what you want from them and write it down. Practice saying what you need and why without getting angry. Ask if there is a worker at the agency who works with young parents. Take a friend with you if you feel worried.

> **☞ Remember!!**
>
> • Be wise enough to learn from others.
>
> • Be smart enough to say, "I don't know."
>
> • Get lots of information so you have plenty of ideas to make good choices.
>
> • Everyone is allowed to make mistakes; mistakes are to learn from.
>
> • Use the "survival instinct" strengths that you develop as a young parent.
>
> • Find support for yourself and use it.
>
> • Do not be ashamed to ask for help.

Be willing to listen to family members when they give advice. The more ideas you get, the more ideas you have to choose from. It does not mean you have to follow the advice. Choose what feels right for you.

Ask workers you trust for referrals to people they know who will be able to help you.

Part Three

Staying Healthy During Your Pregnancy

Chapter 11

Having A Healthy Pregnancy

If you're a pregnant teen, you're not alone. About half a million adolescents give birth each year. Most teens who have babies didn't plan on becoming pregnant. You may have been surprised when you found out or even hoped it wasn't true. You may have been terrified to tell your parents. You may have worried how this might affect your relationships with your family, friends, and the baby's father. Sharing the news of your pregnancy can be one of the most difficult conversations to have.

Whether you feel confused, worried, scared, or excited, you'll want to know how your life will change, what you can do to have a healthy baby, and what it takes to become a good parent.

The most important thing you can do is to take good care of yourself so that you and your baby will be healthy.

Prenatal Care

If you are pregnant, you need to see a doctor as soon as possible to begin getting prenatal care (medical care during pregnancy). The sooner you start to get medical care, the better your chances that you and your baby will be healthy.

About This Chapter: This information was provided by KidsHealth, one of the largest resources online for medically reviewed health information written for parents, kids, and teens. For more articles like this one, visit www.KidsHealth.org, or www.TeensHealth.org. © 2004 The Nemours Foundation.

During your first visit, your doctor will
ask you lots of questions including the
date of your last period. This is so he
or she can estimate how long you have
been pregnant and your due date. Doctors measure pregnancies in weeks. It's
important to remember that your due date
is only an estimate: Most babies are born be-
tween 38 and 42 weeks after the first day of a woman's last menstrual period,
or 36 to 38 weeks after conception (when the sperm fertilizes the egg). Only
a small percentage of women actually deliver exactly on their due dates.

♣ It's A Fact!!

Girls who get the proper care
and make the right choices have
a very good chance of having
healthy babies.

A pregnancy is divided into three phases, or trimesters. The first trimester is from conception to the end of week 13. The second trimester is from
week 14 to the end of week 26. The third trimester is from week 27 to the
end of the pregnancy.

The doctor will examine you and perform a pelvic exam. He or she will
also perform blood tests, a urine test, and tests for sexually transmitted diseases (STDs), including a test for HIV, which is on the rise in teens. (Some
STDs can cause serious medical problems in newborns, so it's important to
get treatment to protect the baby.)

The doctor will explain the types of physical and emotional changes you
can expect during pregnancy. He or she will also teach you how to recognize
the signs of possible problems during pregnancy (called complications). This
is especially important because teens are more at risk for certain complications such as anemia, high blood pressure, miscarriage, and delivering a baby
earlier than usual (called premature delivery).

✔ Quick Tip

If you can't afford to go to a doctor or clinic for prenatal care,
there are social service organizations that can help you. Ask your
parent, school counselor, or another trusted adult to help
you locate resources in your community.

Your doctor will want you to start taking prenatal vitamins that contain the minerals folic acid, calcium, and iron as soon as possible. The vitamins may be prescribed by the doctor, or he or she may recommend a brand that you can buy over the counter. These vitamins and minerals help ensure the baby's and mother's health as well as prevent some types of birth defects.

Ideally, you should see your doctor once each month for the first 28 to 30 weeks of your pregnancy, then every two to three weeks until 36 weeks, then once a week until you deliver the baby. If you have a medical condition such as diabetes that needs careful monitoring during your pregnancy, your doctor will probably want to see you more often.

> ✔ **Quick Tip**
>
> One part of prenatal care is attending classes where expectant mothers can learn about having a healthy pregnancy and delivery and the basics of caring for a new baby. These classes may be offered at hospitals, medical centers, schools, and colleges in your area.

During visits, your doctor will check your weight, blood pressure, and urine, and will measure your abdomen to keep track of the baby's growth. Once the baby's heartbeat can be heard with a special device, the doctor will listen for it at each visit. Your doctor will probably also send you for some other tests during the pregnancy, such as an ultrasound, to make sure that everything is OK with your baby.

It can be difficult for adults to talk to their doctors about their bodies and even more difficult for teens to do so. Your doctor is there to help you stay healthy during pregnancy and to have a healthy baby—and there's probably not much he or she hasn't heard from expectant mothers. So don't be afraid to ask questions. Think of your doctor both as a resource and a friend who you can confide in about what's happening to you. And always be honest when your doctor asks questions about issues that could affect your baby's health.

Changes To Expect In Your Body

Pregnancy causes lots of physical changes in the body. Here are some common ones.

Breast Growth: An increase in breast size is one of the first signs of pregnancy, and the breasts may continue to grow throughout the pregnancy. You may go up several bra sizes during the course of your pregnancy.

Skin Changes: Don't be surprised if people tell you your skin is "glowing" when you are pregnant—pregnancy causes an increase in blood volume, which can make your cheeks a little pinker than usual. And hormonal changes increase oil gland secretion, which can give your skin a shinier appearance. Acne is also common during pregnancy for the same reason.

Other skin changes caused by pregnancy hormones may include brownish or yellowish patches on the face called chloasma and a dark line on the midline of the lower abdomen, known as the linea nigra.

Also, moles or freckles that you had prior to pregnancy may become bigger and darker. Even the areola, the area around the nipples, becomes darker. Stretch marks are thin pink or purplish lines that can appear on your abdomen, breasts, or thighs.

Except for the darkening of the areola, which is usually permanent, these skin changes will usually disappear after you give birth.

Mood Swings: It's very common to have mood swings during pregnancy. Some girls may also experience depression during pregnancy or after delivery. If you have symptoms of depression such as sadness, changes in sleep patterns, or bad feelings about yourself or your life for more than two weeks, tell your doctor so he or she can help you to get treatment.

Pregnancy Discomforts: Pregnancy can cause some uncomfortable side effects. These include nausea and vomiting, especially early in the pregnancy; leg swelling; varicose veins in the legs and the area around the vaginal opening; hemorrhoids; heartburn and constipation; backache; fatigue; and sleep loss. If you experience one or more of these side effects, keep in mind that you're not alone. Ask your doctor for advice on how to deal with these common problems.

Things To Avoid

Smoking, drinking, and taking drugs when you are pregnant put you and your baby at risk for a number of serious problems.

Alcohol: Doctors now feel that it's not safe to drink any amount of alcohol when you are pregnant. Drinking can harm a developing fetus, putting a baby at risk for birth defects and mental problems.

Smoking: The risks of smoking during pregnancy include stillbirths (when a baby dies while inside the mother), low birth weight (which increases a baby's risk for health problems), prematurity (when babies are born earlier than 37 weeks), and sudden infant death syndrome (SIDS). SIDS is the sudden, unexplained death of an infant who is younger than one year old.

Drugs: Using illegal drugs such as cocaine or marijuana during pregnancy can cause miscarriage, prematurity, and other medical problems. Babies can also be born addicted to certain drugs.

Ask your doctor for help if you are having trouble quitting smoking, drinking, or drugs. Check with your doctor before taking any medication while you are pregnant, including over-the-counter medications, herbal remedies and supplements, and vitamins.

Unsafe Sex: Talk to your doctor about sex during pregnancy. If you are sexually active while you are pregnant, you must use a condom to help prevent getting an STD. Some STDs can cause blindness, pneumonia, or meningitis in newborns, so it's important to protect yourself and your baby.

Taking Care Of Yourself During Pregnancy

Eating: Many girls worry about how their bodies look and are afraid to gain weight during pregnancy. But now that you are eating for two, this is not a good time to cut calories or go on a diet. Don't try to hide your pregnancy by dieting—both you and your baby need certain nutrients to grow properly. Eating a variety of healthy foods, drinking plenty of water, and cutting back on high-fat junk foods will help you and your developing baby to be healthy.

Doctors generally recommend adding about 250 calories a day to your diet to provide adequate nourishment for the developing fetus. Depending on your prepregnancy weight, you should gain about 25 to 35 pounds during pregnancy, most of this during the last six months. Your doctor will advise you about this based on your individual situation.

Eating additional fiber—20 to 30 grams a day—and drinking plenty of water can help to prevent common problems such as constipation. Good sources of fiber are fresh fruits and vegetables and whole-grain breads, cereals, or muffins.

Exercise: Exercising during pregnancy is good for you as long as you choose appropriate activities. Doctors generally recommend low-impact activities such as walking, swimming, and yoga. Contact sports and high-impact aerobic activities that pose a greater risk of injury should generally be avoided. Also, working at a job that involves heavy lifting is not recommended for women during the last trimester of pregnancy. Talk to your doctor if you have questions about whether particular types of exercise are safe for you and your baby.

Sleep: It's important to get plenty of rest while you are pregnant. Early in your pregnancy, try to get into the habit of sleeping on your side. Lying on your side with your knees bent is likely to be the most comfortable position as your pregnancy progresses. Also, it makes your heart's job easier because it keeps the baby's weight from applying pressure to the large vein that carries blood back to the heart from your feet and legs.

Some doctors specifically recommend that girls who are pregnant sleep on the left side. Because your liver is on the right side of your abdomen, lying on your left side helps keep the uterus off that large organ. Ask what your doctor recommends—in most cases, lying on either side should do the trick and help take some pressure off your back.

Stress can interfere with sleep. Maybe you're worried about your baby's health, about delivery, or about what your new role as a parent will be like. All of these feelings are normal, but they may keep you up at night. Talk to your doctor if you are having problems sleeping during your pregnancy.

Emotional Health: It's common for pregnant teens to feel a range of emotions, such as fear, anger, guilt, and sadness. It may take a while to adjust to the fact that you're going to have a baby. It's a huge change, and it's natural for pregnant teens to wonder whether they're ready to handle the responsibilities that come with being a parent.

How a girl feels often depends on how much support she has from the baby's father, from her family (and the baby's father's family), and from friends. Each girl's situation is different. Depending on your situation, you may need to seek more support from people outside your family. It's important to talk to the people who can support and guide you and help you share and sort through your feelings. Your school counselor or nurse can refer you to resources in your community that can help.

School And The Future

Some girls plan to raise their babies themselves. Sometimes grandparents or other family members help. Some girls decide to give their babies up for adoption. It takes a great deal of courage and concern for the baby to make these difficult decisions.

Girls who complete high school are more likely to have good jobs and enjoy more success in their lives. If possible, finish high school now rather than trying to return later. Ask your school counselor or an adult you trust for information about programs and classes in your community for pregnant teens.

Some communities have support groups especially for teen parents. Some high schools have child care centers on campus. Perhaps a family member or friend can care for your baby while you're in school.

Life takes unexpected turns. These changes often bring opportunities to learn and grow and develop new strengths. You can stay informed by reading books, attending classes, or checking out reputable websites on child raising. Keep communications open in your own family and talk to your parents about this new phase in your life. Your baby's doctor, your parents, family members, or other adults can all help guide you while you are pregnant and when you become a parent.

Chapter 12

Choosing A Health Care Provider For You And Your Baby

Choosing A Caregiver

Why is choosing a caregiver one of the most important maternity decisions I will make?

Early in your pregnancy it is important to make thoughtful decisions about who will be your caregiver and where you plan to give birth. These major decisions can influence the following:

- The care that you receive and the effects of that care

- The quality of your relationship with your main and other caregivers

- The amount of information you receive

- The choices and options you will have, particularly during your labor and birth

- The degree to which you are involved with decisions about your care

About This Chapter: © 2006 Childbirth Connection. Reprinted with permission of Childbirth Connection from "Choosing a Caregiver," http://childbirthconnection.org/article.asp?ck=10158 (accessed November 2006); "Options: Caregiver," http://childbirthconnection.org/article.asp?ck=10163 (accessed November 2006); and "Tips & Tools: Caregiver," http://childbirthconnection.org/article.asp?ck=10160 (accessed November 2006).

It may take some time and energy to find the right caregiver and birth setting. These important decisions are well worth the effort.

How will my choice of caregiver influence where I can give birth?

Caregivers and birth settings usually go hand in hand. As you explore your different options, you will want to decide on a caregiver who practices in a birth setting that will meet your needs. For example, if you decide that you would like to work with a physician, you will probably be limited to giving birth at a hospital. If you choose to work with a midwife, you may have more options since midwives practice in hospitals, birth centers, and homes. Moreover, there may be important differences among hospitals and among birth centers. When choosing a caregiver, it is also important to think about choosing a birth setting that is right for you.

♣ **It's A Fact!!**

If you are a well and healthy childbearing woman (as are most pregnant women in the United States), you can choose a midwife or a doctor as your maternity caregiver.

Source: Reprinted with permission of Childbirth Connection from "Choosing a Caregiver," http://childbirthconnection.org/article.asp?ck=10158 (accessed November 2006).

What are important considerations when choosing a maternity caregiver?

The following are signs of an excellent choice of maternity caregiver:

• The caregiver's practices are consistent with the best available research about safe and effective care.

• The caregiver's practices work with the physiology of pregnancy and birth—your body is finely tuned to do this work. Some actions support this work, while others interfere with it.

• The two of you are able to develop a strong relationship with good communication and mutual trust and respect.

• The caregiver's personal style is compatible with your needs, preferences, and values.

What are some insufficient reasons for choosing a caregiver?

It is not wise to select a caregiver solely because of the following:

- That person practices near your home or workplace. Convenience is nice, but you may need to travel further to find the right person.

- You know someone who worked with that person. Even if recommended by a friend or relative, you will want to be sure that a maternity caregiver's style will meet your needs and values and reflects the best available research.

- That person is a woman, or a man. If you have a preference for caregiver gender, you will want to be sure that that person's maternity philosophy and style of practice match well with your needs and values and with the best available research.

- That person has been your provider for well-woman or primary care. You will want to learn about that person's maternity philosophy and style of practice before making your decision.

How do types of caregivers differ from one another?

In making your decision, keep in mind that caregivers vary in important ways:

- Philosophy of birth and model of care
- Style of practice—includes the amount of time spent with you, interest in sharing information and involving you in decision-making, and preferences for use of interventions
- Birth settings—most caregivers work at one or two sites, few offer the full range of hospital, out-of-hospital birth center, and home birth
- Whether specific types of caregivers are available in your area
- Whether your insurance will cover their services

What if I change my mind and want to switch to another caregiver?

As time goes on, you will learn more about your needs and about the caregiver and birth setting that you have chosen. If you have concerns and have not been able to resolve them through open and respectful communication, you may begin to wonder if you have made the right choice(s). Do not hesitate to explore other options. Even if it is late in your pregnancy, you can switch if the following is true:

> ♣ **It's A Fact!!**
> Several types of midwives and several types of physicians provide prenatal care, attend births, and care for women after birth in the United States.
>
> Source: "Options: Caregiver," http://childbirthconnection.org/article.asp?ck=10163 (accessed November 2006).

- You have enough time to explore options and find a situation that you believe will work better for you.

- The new caregiver or setting has no policies that prevent you from making this change at that time in your pregnancy.

- Your insurance will cover the new arrangements, or you are willing and able to pay out of pocket.

You may have to change your caregiver and/or birth setting to get what you want.

Caregiver Options

What types of caregivers provide maternity care? What are my options?

The great majority of childbearing women in the U.S. is well and healthy and can consider choosing from among the full range of maternity caregivers. If you have a serious medical condition or are at high risk for developing such a condition, you will probably want to (1) be in the care of a doctor who has completed a residency and is board-certified in obstetrics and (2) plan to give birth in a hospital. Maternity caregivers understand and can advise you about situations that may call for more specialized care.

What are the "midwifery model of care" and the "medical model of care"?

Views of the childbearing process and of appropriate care for childbearing women vary. Two contrasting perspectives are often called the "midwifery model of care" and the "medical model of care." There are striking differences in the two models. These differences can have a great impact on your experience and outcomes.

Table 12.1. Midwifery Model of Care Vs. Medical Model of Care

Midwifery Model of Care	Medical Model of Care
Focus on health, wellness, prevention	Focus on managing problems and complications
Labor/birth as normal physiological processes	Labor/birth as dependent on technology
Lower rates of using interventions	Higher rates of using interventions
Mother gives birth	Doctor delivers baby
Care is individualized	Care is routinized

Naturally, the midwifery model describes the practice of many midwives, and the medical model describes the practice of many doctors; but many caregivers combine elements of both. It is possible, but less common, to find doctors whose practice most closely resembles the midwifery model of care and midwives whose practice most closely resembles the medical model.

Thinking about these different views can help you to understand your own values and ideas about pregnancy and birth and can help you select a caregiver who is compatible with your needs and values. Many women have a clear preference for one or the other of these models.

What is a midwife?

Midwives are well suited to care for healthy women who expect to have a normal birth. They provide prenatal care, care during labor and birth, and care after the birth. Many give priority to providing good information to women, involving women in decision-making, and providing flexible and responsive care. Many work to avoid unnecessary tests and treatments, and women under the care of midwives typically are less likely to have a cesarean,

♣ **It's A Fact!!**

Some midwives also have additional training and credentials for childbirth education, breastfeeding consultation, and/or doula care.

Source: "Options: Caregiver," http://childbirthconnection.org/article.asp?ck=10163 (accessed November 2006).

an episiotomy, and other interventions than women receiving care from doctors. Some midwives provide continuous support throughout labor and birth, which has many benefits for women, infants, and families and no known risks. Midwives often encourage, are well informed about, and provide much support for breastfeeding.

Where do midwives practice? What are trends in the use of midwifery care?

Midwives attend births in many hospitals throughout the United States, and they attend most of the births that take place in out-of-hospital birth centers and homes. They provide prenatal care and care after birth in many settings.

At this time, midwives attend about eight percent of births in the U.S.—over 300,000 every year. The trend shows a steady increase in use of midwifery services over time. (In 1975, midwives attended about one percent of U.S. births.) In contrast to the U.S., midwives are the most common maternity caregiver in many countries in Europe and elsewhere.

What types of midwives practice in the U.S.?

Certified Nurse-Midwives (CNMs) are educated in the two disciplines of nursing and midwifery. They are registered nurses who have graduated from a nurse-midwifery education program accredited by the American College of Nurse-Midwives (ACNM). They are "certified" when they pass an exam of the ACNM Certification Council and are licensed by their state to practice nurse-midwifery. All 50 states license CNMs, and most midwives who practice in the U.S. are CNMs.

CNMs are trained to provide prenatal care, care during labor and birth, and follow-up care to the mother and newborn after the birth. Most CNMs attend births in hospitals, but they also attend births in out-of-hospital birth centers and in women's homes. CNMs may also provide "well-woman" care, such as gynecological checkups, pelvic and breast exams, and pap smears, as well as family planning care.

CNMs may work within a midwifery-owned and led practice, in a practice with physicians, or as employees of hospitals, health plans, or public agencies. In all cases, they are required to have established relationships with physicians for consultation, collaboration, and referral, as needed.

Certified Professional Midwives (CPMs) have passed the certification examination of the North American Registry of Midwives (NARM). Candidates for this exam are educated in core content areas, complete a core set of clinical experiences, demonstrate core skills, and present practice plans (including care guidelines and an emergency care plan). The NARM certification process recognizes multiple routes of entry into midwifery, and most CPMs become midwives without first becoming a nurse. Many states in the U.S. license CPMs or legally recognize them in other ways.

The CPM credential requires knowledge of, and experience in, out-of-hospital settings, and most CPMs attend births in women's homes or in out-of-hospital birth centers. They usually do not practice in hospitals. CPMs provide prenatal care, care during labor and birth, and care of the new mother and her baby in the early weeks after birth.

Certified Midwives (CMs) are new professionals in the health care field. The American College of Nurse-Midwives (ACNM) has recently begun to certify midwives who do not also have training in nursing. Although not registered nurses, CMs may have backgrounds as physician assistants, physical therapists, or other health practitioners. CM education closely mirrors the education of certified nurse-midwives, and CMs graduate from an education program accredited by the ACNM. CMs are "certified" when they pass the same exam that the ACNM Certification Council gives to certified nurse-midwives. The settings in which they practice and the care they provide are comparable to CNMs. New York is the only state with CM licensure at this time.

Other Midwives offering home birth services do not have any of the above credentials. State regulatory mechanisms for such midwives vary widely, from recognition to prohibition of their practice. Although they may have considerable education and experience, established arrangements for consulting with and referring to physicians, and other important qualifications for midwifery practice, women who are considering using their services must carefully explore these questions with the midwife.

What are characteristics of medical training and practice for maternity care?

Medical training for maternity care emphasizes expertise in identifying and managing risks and complications. For this reason, doctors who provide maternity care, and especially obstetric specialists, are optimal caregivers for women with serious health problems or risks for such problems.

Because of this focus on problems, medical maternity care may emphasize physical concerns and give less attention to emotional matters or normal childbearing processes. From this perspective, many tests and treatments may be recommended for well women to be sure nothing is wrong or in case a problem may arise. The role of the doctor may be to take charge by managing care and delivering the baby. Rules, restrictions, and routines may be applied to most women.

Where do physicians practice? What are trends in the use of physician care?

Nearly all physician-attended births in the U.S. are in hospitals. A small number of physicians attend births in out-of-hospital birth centers or in homes. They provide prenatal care and care after birth in office settings.

Physicians attend over 90 percent of births in the U.S. at this time. With the growth of midwifery care in the U.S. during the last quarter century, this proportion has been declining.

What types of physicians provide maternity care?

Family Physicians (FPs) are doctors who provide cradle-to-grave care to the whole family and approach care from a family-oriented perspective. They address needs and concerns relating to all bodily systems. This means that they can provide ongoing care for mothers, babies, and other family members.

Roughly 25 percent of family practice physicians provide maternity care and attend births. They may work together with an obstetrician, or refer to an obstetrician, if a complication arises. Quite a few FPs are trained in surgery and perform cesarean sections. A "board-certified" family physician has received an MD or DO degree from an accredited school, completed three years of training and practice in an accredited family practice residency program, and passed an examination given by the American Board of Family Practice. All 50 states license family physicians.

Studies comparing practice styles of family physicians to other maternity caregivers have generally found that women using FPs are more likely than midwives and less likely than obstetricians to have common maternity interventions, such as cesarean section, episiotomy, and labor induction. FPs may combine both an obstetric style of maternity practice and a view of childbirth as an important family event and normal life process. Within family medicine, general family care leads seamlessly to maternity care. And maternity care leads directly into women's postpartum health care, and newborn and baby care.

Obstetricians are doctors who have special training in prenatal care, labor, birth, high-risk pregnancy, and surgery. Many obstetricians also provide gynecological care and other health services to women.

Obstetricians are well suited to care for women with established serious medical problems or who are at high risk for developing such problems. Many obstetricians approach birth as a medical event best managed by highly trained specialists. Obstetricians tend to have higher rates of interventions (such as cesareans and episiotomy) than family physicians and midwives, even when the health status and risk level of women is similar.

Providers who are "board-certified" in obstetrics and gynecology have received an MD or DO degree from an accredited school, completed at least four years of training and practice in an accredited obstetrics and gynecology residency program, and passed an examination given by the American Board of Obstetrics and Gynecology. All 50 states license obstetricians.

Osteopaths (DOs) are graduates of accredited colleges of osteopathic medicine. Osteopathic medicine complements use of medical tests and treatments with hands-on diagnosis and treatment known as "osteopathic manipulative treatment." This approach gives special attention to muscles, bones, and nerves. Nearly all DOs complete residency training in a specialized area of medicine. Osteopaths trained in family medicine or in obstetrics and gynecology may provide maternity care. Osteopaths are "board-certified" in these specialties if they receive the DO degree, complete an accredited residency program, and pass the examination given by the American Board of Family Practice, The American Board of Obstetrics and Gynecology, or the corresponding specialty boards of the American Osteopathic Association. All 50 states license DOs, and they attend about four percent of births in the U.S.

We do not have good information to help us characterize the maternity care practice style of osteopaths. Osteopaths may combine both an obstetric style of maternity practice and a view of childbirth as a normal physiological process.

Tips For Choosing A Caregiver

How can I become familiar with my options before making my decision?

We encourage you to meet with several caregivers to explore options and become informed before making this important decision. If you are unsure about which type of caregiver to work with, you can interview different types of maternity caregivers. If you know you want to work with a specific type of caregiver, it is a good idea to consider more than one individual before making this important decision as personal styles and practices can vary.

What should I ask myself about the experience of meeting with a maternity caregiver?

When you go to interview a caregiver, and during your prenatal visits, ask yourself how you feel about the experience:

- Is this person listening to me and respectful of my wish to make careful decisions?

- Is the person willing to take the time to answer my questions to my satisfaction?

- Does this person share my vision for my maternity care and birth?

- Do I think that I can feel comfortable with and trust this person?

- Can I get what I want from this person?

- Does this feel right for me?

This person will be working intimately with you and your family through one of the most important times of your life. Follow your instincts. Only you can make the decision that is right for you. If you have concerns, even if you are well into your pregnancy and prenatal care, it may be important to explore other options.

How should I go about interviewing possible caregivers?

Make arrangements for a separate visit that is devoted to learning about the caregiver and practice—a "consultation" rather than an "intake" visit. This will give you a chance to gather information before you commit to working with one caregiver or another. Find out in advance whether the office charges for such a visit and, if so, whether your insurance company will pay for a consultation for this purpose. Some practices offer regular informal get-togethers for newly pregnant women to meet with caregivers and learn about the practice.

You may want to ask your partner or a friend to come with you to the interview. This will allow you to discuss your thoughts and impressions afterward with someone you know and trust.

Having a list of questions with you can help, as well as doing the following:

- Organize your thoughts and concerns.

- Ensure that you get all of your questions answered.

- Communicate to the caregiver that you are serious about your needs and preferences and eager to be involved in decisions about your care.

- Show respect for the caregiver's time by being organized and efficient.

- Compare answers from different caregivers.

If you are interested in working with a specific caregiver, it is also important to do the following:

- Meet, and be sure you feel comfortable with, anyone else who may be "on call" to attend your birth, even if practitioners work together in some capacity, their philosophy and approach can differ.

- Explore, and be sure you are comfortable with, the birth setting where the caregiver works; you can usually take a tour.

How do I know that a caregiver practices in line with the best research about safe and effective care for mothers and babies?

Maternity care can vary from one caregiver to another. This chapter can help you understand why it is important to choose a caregiver who practices according to the highest standard of care and can help you recognize such care.

How do I find out which caregivers and services are covered by my insurance plan?

Contact your insurance plan to find out the following:

- Names and contact information for local midwives and physicians who are covered by the plan

- Whether the plan covers care in the setting where you wish to give birth

- Whether there are any maternity services that are not covered

- Whether they will cover visits that allow you to meet with caregivers before making your selection

☞ Remember!!

You will also want to check with your provider and birth setting to be sure that they accept your insurance.

Source: "Tips & Tools: Caregiver," http://
childbirthconnection.org/article.asp?ck=10160
(accessed November 2006).

Chapter 13

Prenatal Care, Tests, And Procedures

Prenatal Care

What is prenatal care?

Prenatal care is the health care you get while you are pregnant. You can take care of yourself and your baby by getting early prenatal care, getting regular prenatal care, and by following your doctor's advice.

Why do I need prenatal care?

Babies of mothers who do not get prenatal care are three times more likely to have a low birth weight and five times more likely to die than those born to mothers who do get care.

Doctors can spot health problems early when they see mothers regularly. This allows doctors to treat them early. Early treatment can cure many problems and prevent others.

I'm pregnant. What should I do or avoid for a healthy baby?

Some things you can do to take care of yourself and the precious life growing inside you include the following:

About This Chapter: This chapter begins with text excerpted from "Prenatal Care," National Women's Health Information Center (NWHIC), U.S. Department of Health and Human Services, April 2006; and continues with "Prenatal Tests And Procedures," excerpted from "Doctors Visits and Tests," NWHIC, January 2006.

- Take a multivitamin or prenatal vitamin with 400 micrograms (mcg) of folic acid every day.

- Eat a healthy diet that includes fruits, vegetables, grains, and calcium-rich foods. Choose foods low in saturated fat.

- Unless your doctor tells you not to, try to be active for 30 minutes most days of the week.

- If you smoke, drink alcohol, or use drugs, stop.

- Ask your doctor before taking any medicine or herbal products. Some are not safe during pregnancy.

- Avoid hot tubs, saunas, and x-rays.

> ✔ **Quick Tip**
>
> **Do not use scented feminine hygiene products.** Pregnant women should avoid scented sprays, sanitary napkins, and bubble bath. These products might irritate your vaginal area and increase your risk of urinary tract infection or yeast infection.
>
> **Do not douche.** Douching can irritate the vagina, force air into the birth canal and increase the risk of infection.
>
> Source: Excerpted from "Pregnancy Dos and Don'ts," National Women's Health Information Center, February 2006.

- If you have a cat, ask your doctor about toxoplasmosis. This infection is caused by a parasite sometimes found in cat feces. When left untreated, toxoplasmosis can cause birth defects.

- Do not eat uncooked or undercooked meats or fish.

- Stay away from chemicals like insecticides, solvents (like some cleaners or paint thinners), lead, and mercury.

- Avoid or control caffeine in your diet. Pregnant women should have no more than two servings of caffeine per day.

How often should I see my doctor during pregnancy?

Your doctor will give you a schedule of all the doctor's visits you should have while pregnant. Most experts suggest you see your doctor about once each month for the first six months of pregnancy, every two weeks for the seventh and eight month of pregnancy, and every week until the baby is born.

If your pregnancy is high risk because of health problems (like diabetes or high blood pressure), you will probably see your doctor more often.

What happens during prenatal visits?

During the first prenatal visit, you can expect your doctor or nurse to do the following:

- ask about your health history including diseases, operations, or prior pregnancies

- ask about your family's health history

- do a complete physical exam

- do a pelvic exam with a Pap test

- order tests of your blood and urine

- check your blood pressure, urine, height, and weight

- figure out your expected due date

- answer your questions

Later prenatal visits will probably be shorter. Most prenatal visits will include checking the baby's heart rate, checking your blood pressure, checking your urine for signs of diabetes, and measuring your weight gain.

While you are pregnant, your doctor or midwife may suggest a number of laboratory tests, ultrasound exams, and other screening tests.

✔ **Quick Tip**

Consider getting a flu shot. The flu can be dangerous for some moms-to-be. The Centers for Disease Control and Prevention (CDC) suggests vaccinations for all women who are at least 14 weeks pregnant during the flu season. Ask your doctor if you should get a flu shot.

Source: Excerpted from "Pregnancy Dos and Don'ts,"
National Women's Health Information
Center, February 2006.

Where can I go to get free or reduced-cost prenatal care?

Women in every state can get help to pay for medical care during their pregnancies. Programs give medical care, information, advice, and other services.

To find out about the program in your state, you can call 800-311-BABY (800-311-2229). This toll-free telephone number will connect you to the health department in your area code. For information in Spanish, call 800-504-7081. You may also call or contact your local health department.

Prenatal Tests And Procedures

Screening Tests

Screening tests measure the risk of having a baby with some genetic birth defects. Birth defects are caused by problems with a baby's genes, inherited factors passed down from the mother and the father. Birth defects can also occur randomly in people with no family history of that disorder.

The benefit of screening tests is that they do not pose any risk to the fetus or mother, but screening tests cannot tell for sure if the baby has a birth defect. Instead, screening tests give the odds of your baby having a birth defect based on your age.

Targeted Ultrasound: The best time to receive this test is between 18 and 20 weeks of pregnancy. Most major problems with the way your baby might be formed can be seen at this time. This test is not the most accurate for finding out whether your baby has Down syndrome. In most cases, your doctor can find out the sex of your baby by using ultrasound.

Maternal Serum Marker Screening Test: This blood test can be called by many different names including multiple marker screening test, triple test, quad screen, and others. This test is usually given between 15 and 20 weeks of pregnancy. It checks for birth defects such as Down syndrome.

Nuchal Translucency Screening (NTS): This screening can be done between 11 and 14 weeks of pregnancy. It uses an ultrasound and blood test to calculate the risk of some birth defects.

Diagnostic Tests

Diagnostic tests can give definite "yes" or "no" answers about whether your baby has a birth defect. But, unlike screening tests, they are invasive or come with a risk of miscarriage. Amniocentesis and chorionic villus sampling (CVS) are the two most commonly used. Both tests are more than 99% accurate for finding these problems. These tests also can tell you your baby's sex.

Amniocentesis: This test is performed in pregnancies of at least 16 weeks. It involves your doctor inserting a thin needle through your abdomen, into your uterus, and into the amniotic sac to take out a small amount of amniotic fluid for testing. The cells from the fluid are grown in a lab to look for problems with chromosomes. About 1 in 200 women have a miscarriage as a result of this test.

Chorionic Villus Sampling (CVS): This test is performed between 10 and 12 weeks of pregnancy. The doctor inserts a needle through your abdomen or inserts a catheter through your cervix in order to reach the placenta. Your doctor then takes a sample of cells from the placenta. These cells are used in a lab to look for problems with chromosomes. About 1 in 200 women have a miscarriage as a result of this test.

Chapter 14

How Your Body Changes During Pregnancy

Body Changes

Aches, Pains, And Backaches

As your uterus expands, pains in the back, abdomen, groin area, and thighs often appear. Many women also have backaches and aching near the pelvic bone due to the pressure of the baby's head, increased weight, and loosening joints.

To ease some of these aches and pains try lying down, resting, and applying heat.

Breast Changes

Hormone changes will cause your breasts to get even bigger in preparation for breastfeeding. Your breasts may feel full and heavy, and they might be tender or uncomfortable.

In the third trimester, some pregnant women begin to leak colostrum from their breasts. Colostrum is the first milk that your breasts produce for the baby. It is a thick, yellowish fluid containing antibodies that protect newborns from infection.

About This Chapter: Information in this chapter is from "Pregnancy Basics," The National Women's Health Information Center, U.S. Department of Health and Human Services, Office On Women's Health, January 2006.

Try the following tips to stay comfortable:

- Wear a soft, comfortable maternity or nursing bra with extra support.

- Wash your nipples with water instead of soap. If you have cracked nipples, use a heavy moisturizing cream that contains lanolin.

> **✔ Quick Tip**
>
> Call your doctor as soon as possible if you faint. Dizziness or lightheadedness can be discussed at regular prenatal visits.

Dizziness

Many pregnant women complain of dizziness and lightheadedness. The growth of more blood vessels in early pregnancy, the pressure of the expanding uterus on blood vessels, and the body's increased need for food all can make a pregnant woman feel lightheaded and dizzy.

To feel better, stand up slowly. When you are feeling lightheaded, lay down on your left side. Avoid sitting or standing in one position for a long time. Eat healthy snacks or small meals frequently. Do not get overheated.

Hemorrhoids

Up to 50% of pregnant women get hemorrhoids. Hemorrhoids are swollen and bulging veins in the rectum. They can cause itching, pain, and bleeding.

During pregnancy there is a huge increase in the amount of blood in the body. This can cause veins to enlarge. The expanding uterus also puts pressure on the veins in the rectum. Plus, constipation can make hemorrhoids worse. Hemorrhoids usually improve after delivery.

To help prevent and relieve hemorrhoids drink lots of fluids and eat plenty of fiber-rich foods like whole grains, raw or cooked leafy green vegetables, and fruits. Try not to strain for bowel movements and talk with your doctor before taking any laxative. You may want to ask your doctor about using witch hazel or ice packs to soothe hemorrhoids.

Leg Cramps

At different times during your pregnancy, you might have cramps in your legs or feet. They usually happen at night. This is due to a change in the way your body processes, or metabolizes, calcium.

Try the following tips to prevent and ease leg cramps:

- Eat lots of low-fat calcium-rich foods.

- Get regular, mild exercise, like walking.

- Ask your doctor if you should be taking a prenatal vitamin containing calcium.

- Gently stretch the muscle to relieve leg and foot cramps. If you have a sudden leg cramp, flex your foot towards your body.

- Use heating pads or warm, moist towels to help relax the muscles and ease leg and foot cramps.

Nasal Problems

Nosebleeds and nasal stuffiness are common during pregnancy. They are caused by the increased amount of blood in your body and hormones acting on the tissues of your nose.

To ease nosebleeds, blow gently when you blow your nose. Stop nosebleeds by squeezing your nose between your thumb and finger for a few minutes. If you have nosebleeds that do not stop in a few minutes, or happen often, see your doctor.

Drinking extra water and using a cool mist humidifier in your bedroom may help relieve nasal stuffiness.

Shortness Of Breath

As the baby grows, your expanding uterus will put pressure on all of your organs, including your lungs. You may notice that you are short of breath or might not be able to catch your breath.

☞ **Remember!!**

Talk with your doctor before taking any over-the-counter or prescription medicines for colds or nasal stuffiness.

To ease breathing take deep, long breaths. Maintain good posture so your lungs have room to expand. Use an extra pillow and try sleeping on your side to breathe easier at night.

Swelling

Most women develop mild swelling in the face, hands, or ankles at some point in their pregnancies. As the due date approaches, swelling often becomes more noticeable. If you have rapid, significant weight gain, or your hands or feet suddenly get very puffy, call your doctor as soon as possible. It could be a sign of high blood pressure called preeclampsia or toxemia.

To keep swelling to a minimum, drink 8 to 10 eight-ounce glasses of fluids (water is best) daily. Avoid caffeine and try to avoid very salty foods. Rest when you can with your feet elevated and ask your doctor about using support hose.

Teeth And Gums Problems

Pregnant women with gum disease are much more likely to have premature babies with low-birth weight. This may result from the transfer of bacteria in the mother's mouth to the baby during pregnancy. The microbes can reach the baby through the placenta (a temporary organ joining the mother and fetus which supplies the fetus with blood and nutrients), through the amniotic fluid (fluid around the fetus), and through the layer of tissues in the mother's stomach.

> **☞ Remember!!**
> Tell your dentist that you are pregnant.

All needed dental work should be managed early, because having urgent treatment during pregnancy can present risks. Interventions can be started to control risks for gum inflammation and disease.

Varicose Veins

During pregnancy there is a huge increase in the amount of blood in the body. This can cause veins to enlarge. Plus, pressure on the large veins behind the uterus causes the blood to slow in its return to the heart. For these reasons, varicose veins in the legs and anus (hemorrhoids) are more common in pregnancy.

Varicose veins look like swollen veins raised above the surface of the skin. They can be twisted or bulging and are dark purple or blue in color. They are found most often on the backs of the calves or on the inside of the leg.

To reduce the chances of varicose veins, avoid tight knee-highs or garters and sit with your legs and feet raised when possible.

Digestive Difficulties

Constipation

Many pregnant women complain of constipation. High levels of hormones in your pregnant body slow down digestion and relax muscles in the bowels leaving many women constipated. Plus, the pressure of the expanding uterus on the bowels boosts the chances for constipation.

Try these tips to stay more regular:

- Eat fiber-rich foods like fresh or dried fruit, raw vegetables, and whole-grain cereals and breads daily.

- Drink eight to ten glasses of water every day.

- Avoid caffeinated drinks (coffee, tea, colas, and some other sodas), since caffeine makes your body lose fluid needed for regular bowel movements.

- Get moving. Mild exercise like walking may also ease constipation.

Heartburn And Indigestion

Almost every pregnant woman experiences indigestion and heartburn. Hormones and the pressure of the growing uterus cause this discomfort. Pregnancy hormones slow down the muscles of the digestive tract, so food tends to move more slowly, and digestion is sluggish. This causes many pregnant women to feel bloated.

Hormones also relax the valve that separates the esophagus from the stomach. This allows food and acids to come back up from the stomach to the esophagus. The food and acid causes the burning feeling of heartburn. As your baby gets bigger, the uterus pushes on the stomach making heartburn more common in later pregnancy.

To prevent and ease indigestion and heartburn, avoid greasy and fried foods. Eat six to eight small meals instead of three large meals and eat slowly. Do not gain more than the recommended amount of weight. Take small sips of milk, or eat small pieces of chipped ice to soothe burning. Ask your doctor if you can take an antacid medicine.

Stretch Marks And Other Skin Changes

Stretch Marks

Worried about the dreaded stretch marks of pregnancy? The good news is that only about half of pregnant women get stretch marks.

Stretch marks are red, pink, or purple streaks in the skin. Most often they appear on the thighs, buttocks, abdomen, and breasts. These scars are caused by the stretching of the skin, and usually appear in the second half of pregnancy.

The color of stretch marks depends on a woman's skin color. They can be pink, reddish brown, or dark brown streaks. While creams and lotions can keep your skin well moisturized, they do not prevent stretch marks from forming. Most stretch marks fade after delivery to very light lines.

Other Skin Changes

Some women notice other skin changes during pregnancy. For many women, the nipples become darker and browner during pregnancy. Many pregnant women also develop a dark line (called the linea nigra) on the skin that runs from the belly button down to the pubic hairline. Blotchy brown pigmentations on the forehead, nose, and cheeks are also common. These spots are called melasma or chloasma and are more common in darker-skinned women. Most of these skin changes are caused by pregnancy hormones and will fade or disappear after delivery.

Tingling And Itching

Tingling and numbness of the fingers and a feeling of swelling in the hands are common during pregnancy. These symptoms are due to swelling of tissues in the narrow passages in your wrists, and they should disappear after delivery.

About 20 percent of pregnant women feel itchy during pregnancy. Usually women feel itchy in the abdomen, but red, itchy palms, and soles of the feet are also common complaints. Pregnancy hormones and stretching skin are probably to blame for most of your discomfort. Usually the itchy feeling goes away after delivery.

To feel better, use thick moisturizing creams instead of lotions and use gentle soaps. Avoid hot showers or baths that can dry your skin and avoid itchy fabrics and clothes. Try not to get overheated. Heat can make the itching worse.

Sleeping Troubles

During your pregnancy, you might feel tired even after you have had a lot of sleep. Many women find they are particularly exhausted in the first trimester. This is your body's way of telling you that you need more rest.

In the second trimester, tiredness is usually replaced with a feeling of well-being and energy; but in the third trimester, exhaustion often sets in again. As you get larger, sleeping may become more difficult. The baby's movements, bathroom runs, and an increase in the body's metabolism might interrupt or disturb your sleep. Leg cramping can also interfere with a good night's sleep.

Try these tips to feel and sleep better:

- When you are tired, get some rest.

- Try to get about eight hours of sleep every night and a short nap during the day.

- If you feel stressed, try to find ways to relax.

- Sleep on your left side. This will relieve pressure on blood vessels that supply oxygen and nutrients to the fetus.

- If you have high blood pressure during pregnancy, always lay on your left side when you are lying down.

- Avoid eating large meals three hours before going to bed.

- Get some mild exercise like walking.

- Avoid long naps during the day.

Chapter 15

Nutrition: What To Eat While Pregnant

What To Eat

What you eat during your pregnancy can affect the health of your growing baby. Eat healthy meals and snacks and take a multivitamin every day.

Do I really need to "eat for two?"

While you are pregnant, you will need additional nutrients to keep you and your baby healthy; but that does not mean you need to eat twice as much. You should only eat an extra 300 calories per day.

Make sure not to restrict your diet during pregnancy. If you do, your unborn baby might not get the right amounts of protein, vitamins, and minerals. Low-calorie diets can break down a pregnant woman's stored fat. This can lead to the production of substances called ketones. Ketones can be found in the mother's blood and urine and are a sign of starvation. Constant production of ketones can result in a mentally retarded child.

How should my diet change now that I'm pregnant?

If you are eating a healthy diet before you become pregnant, you may only need to make a few changes to meet the special nutritional needs of

About This Chapter: Information under the heading "What To Eat" is from "What to Eat While Pregnant," National Women's Health Information Center, U.S. Department of Health and Human Services, Office On Women's Health, April 2006. Additional text from the American Pregnancy Association is cited separately within the chapter.

♣ It's A Fact!!

To get enough nutrients, pregnant women should take
a multivitamin or prenatal vitamin and eat healthy foods from
the four basic food groups every day.

Source: Excerpted from "What to Eat While Pregnant,"
National Women's Health Information Center,
April 2006.

pregnancy. The American Dietetic Association (ADA) recommends that pregnant women eat a total of 2,500 to 2,700 calories every day.

Fruits and Vegetables: Pregnant women should try to eat seven or more servings of fruits and vegetables combined daily. Fruits and vegetables are rich sources of fiber, vitamins, and minerals. Fruits and vegetables with vitamin C help you and your baby to have healthy gums and other tissues. Vitamin C also helps your body to heal wounds and to absorb iron. Fruits and vegetables also add fiber and minerals to your diet and give you energy. Plus, dark green vegetables have vitamin A, iron, and folate, which are important nutrients during pregnancy.

Whole-Grain or Enriched Breads/Cereals: Pregnant women should eat six to nine servings of whole-grain or enriched breads and/or cereals every day. Whole-grain products and enriched products contain iron, B vitamins, minerals, and fiber. Some breakfast cereals are enriched with 100% of the folic acid your body needs every day. Folic acid has been shown to help prevent some serious birth defects.

Dairy Products: Pregnant women should try to eat four or more servings of low-fat or non-fat milk, yogurt, cheese, or other dairy products every day. Dairy products provide the calcium you and your baby need for strong bones and teeth. Dairy products are also great sources of vitamin A and D, protein, and B vitamins. Vitamin A helps growth, fight infection, and vision. Pregnant women need 1,000 milligrams (mg) of calcium each day. If you are 18 or younger, you need 1,300 mg of calcium each day.

✔ Quick Tip

There are some dangers lurking in the food pregnant women eat. Listeria is a dangerous bacterium that can grow even in cold refrigerators. Toxoplasma is a risky parasite found in undercooked meat and unwashed fruits and vegetables. These things can cause serious illness, or even death, to you or your unborn baby. Follow these food tips to help keep you and your baby healthy:

- Do not eat raw or undercooked meat, poultry, fish, or shellfish.

- Do not eat refrigerated pâtés or meat spreads.

- Do not eat hot dogs and luncheon meats unless they are reheated until steaming hot.

- Do not eat soft cheeses like feta, brie, camembert, "blue-veined cheeses," "queso blanco," "queso fresco," or panela unless the label says they are pasteurized or made from pasteurized milk.

- Do not drink raw or unpasteurized milk or eat foods that contain unpasteurized milk.

- Do not eat unwashed fruits and vegetables.

Source: Excerpted from "Food Don'ts Print and Go Guide," Center for Food Safety and Applied Nutrition, U.S. Food and Drug Administration, January 2006.

Proteins: Pregnant women and their growing babies need ten grams of protein more than non-pregnant women. Pregnant women should eat 60 grams of protein every day. Two or more two to three ounce servings of cooked lean meat, fish, or poultry without skin, or two or more one-ounce servings of cooked meat contain about 60 grams of protein. Protein builds muscle, tissue, enzymes, hormones, and antibodies for you and your baby. Protein-rich foods also have B vitamins and iron, which are important for your blood.

What other nutrients do I need for a healthy pregnancy?

Folic Acid: Pregnant women need 400 micrograms (400 mcg) of folic acid every day to help prevent birth defects. Folic acid is important for any woman who could possibly become pregnant. Folic acid is a B vitamin that helps prevent serious birth defects of a baby's brain or spine called neural tube defects. Getting enough folic acid can also help prevent birth defects like cleft lip and congenital heart disease.

Iron: Pregnant women need twice as much iron, 30 mg per day, than other women. The Centers for Disease Control and Prevention

(CDC) recommends that pregnant women start taking a low-dose iron supplement (30 mg/day) or a multivitamin with iron beginning at the time of their first prenatal visit. Pregnant women should also eat lots of iron-rich foods.

Pregnant women need extra iron for the increased amount of blood in their bodies. Iron helps keep your blood healthy. Plus, your baby will store iron in his body to last through the first few months of life.

Calcium: Pregnant women aged 19 to 50 years should get 1,000 mg/day of calcium. Younger pregnant women need 1,300 mg/day. Low-fat or non-fat milk, yogurt, cheese, or other dairy products are great sources of calcium. Eating green leafy vegetables and calcium-fortified foods like orange juice and breakfast cereal can also provide calcium. If your diet is not providing 1,000 mg/day of calcium, talk to your doctor about taking a calcium supplement.

✔ Quick Tip

- Do not eat swordfish, tilefish, king mackerel, shark, raw or uncooked fish or shellfish, or refrigerated uncooked smoked fish.

- Eat up to one serving (six ounces) per week of tuna steaks, canned albacore or chunk white tuna, halibut, and snapper.

- Eat up to two servings (12 ounces) per week of shrimp, crab, clams, oysters, scallops, canned light tuna, salmon, mahi mahi, pollock, catfish, and cod.

- Check before eating fish caught in local waters. State health departments have guidelines on fish from local waters or get local fish advisories at the U.S. Environmental Protection Agency website (www.epa.gov).

Source: Excerpted from "Fish Facts Print and Go Guide," Center for Food Safety and Applied Nutrition, U.S. Food and Drug Administration, April 2006.

Water: Pregnant women should drink at least six eight-ounce glasses of water per day. Plus, pregnant women should drink another glass of water for each hour of activity.

Water plays a key role in your diet during pregnancy. It carries the nutrients from the food you eat to your baby. It also helps prevent constipation, hemorrhoids, excessive swelling, and urinary tract or bladder infections. Drinking enough water, especially in your last trimester, prevents you from becoming dehydrated. Not getting enough water can lead to premature or early labor.

Should I eat fish when I'm pregnant?

Fish and shellfish can be part of a healthy diet. They are a great source of protein and heart-healthy omega-3 fatty acids, but almost all fish and shellfish contain a harmful substance called mercury.

Eating For Two: Weight Influences On Pregnancy

Text under this heading is reprinted with permission from the American Pregnancy Association, http://www.americanpregnancy.org, © 2006. All rights reserved.

Weight gain during pregnancy helps your baby grow. Gaining weight at a steady rate within recommended boundaries can also lower your chance of having hemorrhoids, varicose veins, stretch marks, backache, fatigue, indigestion, and shortness of breath during pregnancy.

Why is weight gain important during pregnancy?

The extra weight you gain during pregnancy provides nourishment to your developing baby and is also stored for breastfeeding your baby after delivery.

Where does all the extra weight go?

Here is an approximate breakdown of your weight gain:

- Baby: 7–8 pounds
- Placenta: 1–2 pounds
- Amniotic fluid: 2 pounds

- Uterus: 2 pounds

- Maternal breast tissue: 2 pounds

- Maternal blood: 4 pounds

- Fluids in maternal tissue: 4 pounds

- Maternal fat and nutrient stores: 7 pounds

How much total weight should I gain?

The amount of weight you should gain depends on your weight before pregnancy. You should gain as follows:

- 25–35 pounds: If you were a healthy weight before pregnancy.

- 28–40 pounds: If you were underweight before pregnancy.

- 15–25 pounds: If you were overweight before pregnancy.

At what rate should I gain weight during my pregnancy?

How much you should gain depends on your weight before you were pregnant and how far along you are in your pregnancy.

- **Healthy Weight Before Pregnancy:**

  - 3–5 pounds during the first trimester

  - approximately 1–2 pounds per week in the second trimester

  - approximately 1–2 pounds per week in the third trimester

- **Underweight Before Pregnancy:**

  - 5–6 pounds or more in your first trimester; this also can depend on how underweight you were before pregnancy and your health care provider's recommendations

  - 1–2 pounds per week in the second and third trimesters

- **Overweight Before Pregnancy:**

  - approximately 1–2 pounds in the first trimester

  - approximately 1 pound per week during the last six months

♣ It's A Fact!!
What If I Am Carrying Twins?

If you are pregnant with twins, your appropriate weight gain should be monitored by your health care provider. Weight gain should increase significantly (35–45 pounds) but will not double.

Source: Reprinted with permission from the American Pregnancy Association, http://www.americanpregnancy.org, © 2006. All rights reserved.

The goal is to keep weight gain as steady as possible because your baby requires a daily supply of nutrients throughout your pregnancy that comes from what you eat. It is okay for your weight gain to fluctuate a little from week to week. However, you should contact your health care provider if you suddenly gain or lose weight, especially in your third trimester. This could be a sign of preeclampsia.

Does being underweight pose any risks to my baby or me?

Due to morning sickness, many women have trouble gaining weight in the first trimester and worry about what effects this has on their baby's development. Some women loose a little weight in the beginning of their pregnancy. Fortunately, at this time the baby does not need as many calories and nutrients as later in pregnancy. It is important to gain weight at a steady pace throughout pregnancy. If a woman does not gain weight throughout pregnancy, complications such as a low-birth weight infant or premature delivery could occur. Babies who are born to mothers who do not gain more than 20 pounds are often considered small for gestational age (SGA), meaning they may have been malnourished during pregnancy.

How can I eat healthy during my pregnancy?

A sensible meal plan that is rich in vitamins and minerals are essential for a developing baby. You may want to ask your health care provider for food recommendations or seek the help of a dietitian in your area.

Women who are underweight during pregnancy tend to eat low-calorie foods and not enough protein. The following are ways to get more calories:

- Eat breakfast every day. Peanut butter or a slice of cheese on toast can give you an extra protein boost.

- Snack between meals. Yogurt and dried fruits can provide protein, calcium, and minerals.

- Try to eat a little more food each day that are high in good fats such as nuts, fatty fish, avocados, and olive oil.

- Drink juices that are high in vitamin C or beta-carotene, such as grapefruit juice, orange juice, papaya nectar, apricot nectar, and carrot juice.

- Avoid junk food.

- Consult your health care provider about taking prenatal vitamins.

Can gaining too much weight be harmful?

The following are potential problems with gaining too much weight:

- gestational diabetes
- backaches
- leg pain
- increased fatigue
- varicose veins
- increased risk of cesarean delivery
- high blood pressure

How does being obese affect my pregnancy?

Most overweight women have healthy pregnancies and deliver without complications.

However, it is important to be aware of the potential risks that extra weight can have. Pregnant women who are struggling with obesity may have the following:

- an increased risk for gestational diabetes and high blood pressure

- difficulty with hearing the heartbeat and measuring the size of the uterus

- difficulty with vaginal delivery if the fetus is much larger than average

Fortunately, appropriate medical and self-care can lower the risks of these complications. Your health care provider may suggest that more tests be done during pregnancy. These might include ultrasounds to measure your baby's size, glucose tolerance test to screen for gestational diabetes, and other diagnostic tests later in pregnancy to monitor your baby's development.

The following self-care tips are ways you can make your pregnancy a healthy one for you and your baby:

- Avoid pregnancy risks such as alcohol and smoking.

- Try not to gain too much weight. Your health care provider will provide recommended weight gain.

- Be selective about your food choices. Choose food sources that contain vitamins, minerals, and protein.

Chapter 16

Exercise During Pregnancy

Why exercise during pregnancy?

Whether you are pregnant or not, exercise is one of the best things you can do for your physical and emotional health. The American College of Obstetricians and Gynecologists (ACOG) recommends that pregnant women without health problems or pregnancy complications exercise moderately for 30 minutes or more on most, if not all, days of the week.

Pregnant or not, exercise helps keep the heart, bones, and mind healthy. Staying active also seems to give some special added paybacks for pregnant women.

Here are some really good reasons to get regular exercise during pregnancy:

- It can ease and prevent aches and pains of pregnancy including constipation, varicose veins, backaches, and exhaustion.

- Active women seem to be better prepared for labor and delivery and recover more quickly.

- Exercise may lower the risk of high blood pressure and diabetes during pregnancy.

About This Chapter: Information in this chapter is from "Have a Fit Pregnancy," National Women's Health Information Center, U.S. Department of Health and Human Services, January 2006.

- Fit women have an easier time getting back to a healthy weight after delivery.

- Regular exercise may improve sleep during pregnancy.

- Staying active can protect your emotional health. Pregnant women who exercise seem to have better self-esteem and a lower risk of depression and anxiety.

Is exercise safe for all pregnant women?

No, but for most healthy moms-to-be who do not have any pregnancy-related problems, exercise is a safe and valuable habit. Even so, before exercising during pregnancy talk to your doctor or midwife. She will be able to suggest a fitness plan that is safe for you. Getting a doctor's advice is important for both women who exercise before pregnancy and for those who would like to start a fitness routine.

Women with the follow problems may not be able to exercise during pregnancy:

- heart disease

- lung disease

- obesity

- severe diabetes

- thyroid disease

- seizure disorder

- persistent bleeding in the second or third trimester

- complications with past pregnancies

- premature labor

- pregnancy-related high blood pressure

What type of exercise is best during pregnancy?

Low-impact exercise that requires moderate exertion is probably best. Walking, swimming, dancing, and cycling seem to be comfortable and enjoyable activities for most pregnant women.

According to the ACOG, many different types of exercise can be safe for most pregnant women. They do recommend following these guidelines when choosing a pregnancy exercise plan:

- Avoid activities in which you can get hit in the abdomen like kickboxing, soccer, basketball, or ice hockey.

- Steer clear of activities in which you can fall like horseback riding, downhill skiing, and gymnastics.

- Do not scuba dive during pregnancy. Scuba diving can create gas bubbles in your baby's blood that can cause many health problems.

What guidelines should I follow?

Follow these tips to have safe and healthy workouts:

- When you exercise, start slowly, progress gradually, and cool down slowly.

- You should be able to talk while exercising. If not, you may be exercising too intensely.

- Take frequent breaks.

- Do not exercise on your back after the first trimester. This can put too much pressure on an important vein, and limit blood flow to the baby.

- Avoid jerky, bouncing, and high-impact movements. Connective tissues stretch much more easily during pregnancy, so these types of movements put you at risk of joint injury.

- Do not exercise at high altitudes (more than 6,000 feet). It can prevent your baby from getting enough oxygen.

- Make sure you drink lots of fluids before, during, and after exercising.

- Do not work out in extreme heat or humidity.

- If you feel uncomfortable, short of breath, or tired, take a break, and take it easier when you resume exercise.

How will I know if I am overdoing it?

Stop exercising, and call your doctor as soon as possible, if you have any of the following:

- dizziness

- headache

- chest pain

- calf pain or swelling

- abdominal pain

- blurred vision

- fluid leaking from the vagina

- vaginal bleeding

- decreased fetal movement

- contractions

> ✔ **Quick Tip**
>
> **How To Do Kegel Exercises**
>
> Tighten the pelvic floor muscles for 5 to 10 seconds, and then relax for 5 seconds. Repeat 10 to 20 times, 3 times a day. You can do Kegel exercises standing, sitting, or lying down.

How can I prepare my body for labor and delivery?

Pelvic floor exercises, or Kegel exercises, can help prepare your body for delivery. The pelvic floor muscles support the rectum, vagina, and urethra in the pelvis. Strengthening these muscles by doing Kegel exercises may help you have an easier birth. They will also help you avoid leaking urine during and after pregnancy.

Pelvic muscles are the same ones used to stop the flow of urine. Still, it can be hard to find the right muscles to squeeze. You can be sure you are exercising the right muscles, if when you squeeze them, you stop urinating; or you can put a finger into the vagina and squeeze. If you feel pressure around the finger, you have found the pelvic floor muscles.

Chapter 17

Sleeping During Pregnancy

Many expectant parents know how hard it might be to get a good night's sleep in the months that follow the birth of their child, but who would have guessed that catching some ZZZs during pregnancy would prove to be so difficult?

Actually, you may sleep more than usual during the first trimester of your pregnancy. It's normal to feel tired as your body works to protect and nurture the developing baby. The placenta (the organ that nourishes the fetus until birth) is just forming, your body is making more blood, and your heart is pumping faster.

It's usually later in pregnancy, though, that most women have trouble getting enough deep, uninterrupted sleep.

Why Is Sleeping Sometimes Difficult During Pregnancy?

The first and most pressing reason behind sleep problems during pregnancy is the increasing size of the fetus, which can make it hard to find a comfortable sleeping position. If you've always been a back or stomach sleeper, it may be difficult to get used to sleeping on your side (as doctors recom-

About This Chapter: This information was provided by KidsHealth, one of the largest resources online for medically reviewed health information written for parents, kids, and teens. For more articles like this one, visit www.KidsHealth.org, or www.TeensHealth.org. © 2004 The Nemours Foundation.

mend). Also, shifting around in bed becomes more difficult as the pregnancy progresses and your size increases.

Other common physical symptoms may interfere with sleep as well:

- **The frequent urge to urinate:** Your kidneys are working harder to filter the increased volume of blood (30% to 50% more blood than you had before pregnancy) moving through your body, and this filtering process results in more urine. Also, as your baby grows and the uterus gets bigger, the pressure on your bladder increases. This means more trips to the bathroom, day and night. The number of nighttime trips may be greater if your baby is particularly active at night.

- **Increased heart rate:** Your heart rate increases during pregnancy to pump more blood, and as more of your blood supply goes to the uterus, your heart will be working harder to send sufficient blood to the rest of your body.

- **Shortness of breath:** Breathing may feel more difficult as your enlarging uterus takes up more space, resulting in pressure against your diaphragm (the muscle just below your lungs). At the same time, you may notice that you're breathing faster and more deeply, mainly because of increased oxygen needs.

- **Leg cramps and backaches:** Pains in your legs or back are caused by the extra weight you're carrying.

- **Heartburn and constipation:** Many women experience heartburn, which occurs when the stomach contents reflux back up into the esophagus. During pregnancy, the entire digestive system slows down and food tends to remain in the stomach and intestines longer, which may cause heartburn or constipation.

Your sleep problems may have other causes as well. Many pregnant women report that their dreams become more vivid than usual, and some even experience nightmares. Stress can interfere with sleep, too. Maybe you're worried about your baby's health, anxious about your abilities as a parent, or feeling nervous about the delivery itself. All of these feelings are normal, but they may keep you (and your partner) up at night.

✔ Quick Tip
Tips For Sleeping Success

Although they might seem appealing when you're feeling desperate to get some ZZZs, remember that over-the-counter sleep aids, including herbal remedies, are not recommended for pregnant women. Instead, the following pointers may safely improve your chances of getting a good night's sleep:

- Cut out caffeinated drinks like soda, coffee, and tea from your diet as much as possible. Restrict any intake of them to the morning or early afternoon.

- Avoid drinking a lot of fluids or eating a full meal within a few hours of going to bed at night. (But make sure that you also get plenty of nutrients and liquids throughout the day.) Some women find it helpful to eat more at breakfast and lunch and then have a smaller dinner. If nausea is keeping you up, you may want to eat a few crackers before you go to bed.

- Get into a routine of going to bed and waking up at the same time each day.

- Avoid rigorous exercise right before you go to bed. Instead, do something relaxing, like soaking in a warm bath for 15 minutes or having a warm, caffeine-free drink, such as milk with honey or a cup of herbal tea.

- If a leg cramp awakens you, it may help to press your feet hard against the wall or to stand on the leg. Also, make sure that you're getting enough calcium in your diet, which can help reduce leg cramps.

- Take a class in yoga or learn other relaxation techniques to help you unwind after a busy day. (Be sure to discuss any new activity or fitness regimen with your doctor first.)

- If fear and anxiety are keeping you awake, consider enrolling in a childbirth or parenting class. More knowledge and the company of other pregnant women may help to ease the fears that are keeping you awake at night.

Finding A Good Sleeping Position

Early in your pregnancy, try to get into the habit of sleeping on your side. Lying on your side with your knees bent is likely to be the most comfortable position as your pregnancy progresses. It also makes your heart's job easier because it keeps the baby's weight from applying pressure to the large vein (called the inferior vena cava) that carries blood back to the heart from your feet and legs.

Some doctors specifically recommend that pregnant women sleep on the left side. Because your liver is on the right side of your abdomen, lying on your left side helps keep the uterus off that large organ. Ask what your doctor recommends—in most cases, lying on either side should do the trick and help take some pressure off your back.

But don't drive yourself crazy worrying that you might roll over onto your back during the night. Shifting positions is a natural part of sleeping that you can't control. Most likely, during the third trimester of your pregnancy, your body won't shift into the back-sleeping position anyway because it will be too uncomfortable.

If you do shift onto your back and the baby's weight presses on your inferior vena cava, the discomfort will probably wake you up. See what your doctor recommends about this; he or she may suggest that you use a pillow to keep yourself propped up on one side.

Try experimenting with pillows to discover a comfortable sleeping position. Some women find that it helps to place a pillow under their abdomen or between their legs. Also, using a bunched-up pillow or rolled-up blanket at the small of your back may help to relieve some pressure. In fact, you'll find that there are many "pregnancy pillows" on the market. If you're thinking about purchasing one, talk with your doctor first about which one might work for you.

What To Do When You Can't Sleep

Of course, there are bound to be times when you just can't sleep. Instead of tossing and turning, worrying that you're not asleep, and counting the hours until your alarm clock will go off, get up and do something: read a book, listen to music, watch TV, catch up on letters or e-mail, or pursue some other activity you enjoy. Eventually, you'll probably feel tired enough to get back to sleep.

And if possible, take short naps (30 to 60 minutes) during the day to make up for lost sleep. It won't be long before your baby will be setting the sleep rules in your house, so you may as well get used to sleeping in spurts.

Chapter 18

Depression During And After Pregnancy

What is depression?

Depression can be described as feeling sad, blue, unhappy, miserable, or down in the dumps. Most of us feel this way at one time or another for short periods; but true clinical depression is a mood disorder in which feelings of sadness, loss, anger, or frustration interfere with everyday life for an extended time.

How common is depression during and after pregnancy?

Depression that occurs during pregnancy, or within a year after delivery, is called perinatal depression. Often, the depression is not recognized or treated, because some normal pregnancy changes cause similar symptoms and are happening at the same time. Tiredness, problems sleeping, stronger emotional reactions, and changes in body weight may occur during pregnancy and after pregnancy; but these symptoms may also be signs of depression.

What causes depression?

Hormone changes or a stressful life event, such as a death in the family, can cause chemical changes in the brain that lead to depression. Depression is also an illness that runs in some families. Other times, it is not clear what causes depression.

About This Chapter: Information in this chapter is from "Pregnant and Depressed?" National Women's Health Information Center, U.S. Department of Health and Human Services, January 2006.

During Pregnancy: During pregnancy, there are some factors that may increase a woman's chance of depression such as history of depression or substance abuse, family history of mental illness, little support from family and friends, anxiety about the fetus, problems with a previous pregnancy or birth, marital or financial problems, or the young age of the mother.

After Pregnancy: Depression after pregnancy is called postpartum depression or peripartum depression. After pregnancy, hormonal changes in a woman's body may trigger symptoms of depression. During pregnancy, the amount of two female hormones, estrogen and progesterone, in a woman's body increases greatly. In the first 24 hours after childbirth, the amount of these hormones rapidly drops back down to their normal non-pregnant levels.

Other factors that may contribute to postpartum depression include the following:

- Feeling tired after delivery, broken sleep patterns, and not enough rest often keeps a new mother from regaining her full strength for weeks.

- Feeling overwhelmed with a new baby to take care of and doubting your ability to be a good mother.

- Feeling stress from changes in routines. Sometimes, women think they have to be "super mom" or perfect, which is not realistic and can add stress.

- Having feelings of loss—loss of identity of who you are, or were, before having the baby, loss of control, loss of your pre-pregnancy figure, and feeling less attractive.

- Having less free time and less control over time. Having to stay home indoors for longer periods of time and having less time to spend with the your partner and loved ones.

What are warning signs of depression?

Any of these symptoms during and after pregnancy that last longer than two weeks are signs of depression:

- feeling restless or irritable

- feeling sad, hopeless, and overwhelmed

- crying a lot

- having no energy or motivation

- eating too little or too much

- sleeping too little or too much

- trouble focusing, remembering, or making decisions

- feeling worthless and guilty

- loss of interest or pleasure in activities

- withdrawal from friends and family

- having headaches, chest pains, heart palpitations (the heart beating fast and feeling like it is skipping beats), or hyperventilation (fast and shallow breathing)

After pregnancy, signs of depression may also include being afraid of hurting the baby or oneself and not having any interest in the baby.

What's the difference between "baby blues," postpartum depression, and postpartum psychosis?

The baby blues can happen in the days right after childbirth and normally go away within a few days to a week. A new mother can have sudden mood swings, sadness, crying spells, loss of appetite, sleeping problems, and feel irritable, restless, anxious, and lonely. Symptoms are not severe and treatment is not needed, but there are things you can do to feel better. Nap when the baby does. Ask for help from your partner, family members, and friends. Join a support group of new moms, or talk with other moms.

Postpartum depression can happen anytime within the first year after childbirth. A woman may have a number of symptoms such as sadness, lack of energy, trouble concentrating, anxiety, and feelings of guilt and worthlessness. Postpartum depression needs to be treated by a doctor. Counseling, support groups, and medicines are things that can help.

What should I do if I show signs of depression during or after pregnancy?

Here are some helpful tips:

- Try to get as much rest as you can. Try to nap when the baby naps.

- Stop putting pressure on yourself to do everything. Do as much as you can and leave the rest.

- Ask for help with household chores and nighttime feedings. If you can, have a friend or family member help you in the home for part of the day.

> ♣ **It's A Fact!!**
>
> The difference between postpartum depression and the baby blues is that postpartum depression often affects a woman's well-being and keeps her from functioning well for a longer period of time.

- Talk to your partner, family, and friends about how you are feeling.

- Do not spend a lot of time alone. Get dressed and leave the house. Run an errand or take a short walk.

- Talk with other mothers so you can learn from their experiences.

- Join a support group for women with depression. Call a local hotline or look in your telephone book for information and services.

- Do not make any major life changes during pregnancy. Major changes can cause unneeded stress. Sometimes big changes cannot be avoided. When that happens, try to arrange support and help in your new situation ahead of time.

How is depression treated?

There are two common types of treatment for depression. They are as follows:

- **Talk therapy:** This involves talking to a therapist, psychologist, or social worker to learn to change how depression makes you think, feel, and act.

• **Medicine:** Your doctor can give you an antidepressant medicine to help you. These medicines can help relieve the symptoms of depression.

Women who are pregnant or breastfeeding should talk with their doctors about the advantages and risks of taking antidepressant medicines. A mother's depression can affect her baby's development, so getting treatment is important for both mother and baby. The risks of taking medicine have to be weighed against the risks of depression.

Can untreated depression harm my baby?

Depression not only hurts the mother, but also affects her family. Some women with depression have difficulty caring for themselves during pregnancy. They may have trouble eating and will not gain enough weight during the pregnancy; have trouble sleeping; may miss prenatal visits; may not follow medical instructions; have a poor diet; or may use harmful substances, like tobacco, alcohol, or illegal drugs.

Postpartum depression can affect a mother's ability to parent. She may lack energy, have trouble concentrating, be irritable, and not be able to meet her child's needs for love and affection. As a result, she may feel guilty and lose confidence in herself as a mother, which can worsen the depression. It helps if another caregiver can assist in meeting the needs of the baby while mom is depressed.

♣ **It's A Fact!!**

Researchers believe that postpartum depression can affect the infant by causing delays in language development, problems with emotional bonding to others, behavioral problems, lower activity levels, sleep problems, and distress.

Chapter 19

Using Medications During Pregnancy

Is it safe to take medicine while you are pregnant?

Most of the time, medicine a pregnant woman is taking does not enter the fetus, but sometimes it can, causing damage or birth defects. The risk of damage being done to a fetus is the greatest in the first few weeks of pregnancy when major organs are developing, but researchers also do not know if taking medicines during pregnancy also will have negative effects on the baby later.

Many drugs that you can buy over-the-counter (OTC) in drug and discount stores, and drugs your health care provider prescribes, are thought to be safe to take during pregnancy, although there are no medicines that are proven to be absolutely safe when you are pregnant. Many of these products tell you on the label if they are thought to be safe during pregnancy. If you are not sure you can take an OTC product, ask your health care provider.

Some drugs are not safe to take during pregnancy. Even drugs prescribed to you by your health care provider before you became pregnant might be harmful to both you and the growing fetus during pregnancy. Make sure all of your health care providers know you are pregnant, and never take any drugs during pregnancy unless they tell you to.

About This Chapter: Information in this chapter is from "Pregnancy and Medications," National Women's Health Information Center, U.S. Department of Health and Human Services, November 2002. Updated January 2007 by David A. Cooke, M.D., Diplomate, American Board of Internal Medicine.

♣ It's A Fact!!
Acne Treatment During Pregnancy

During pregnancy, elevated hormone levels can bring a variety of skin changes, including acne. Acne can be treated by a dermatologist in non-pregnant women through prescription drugs such as Accutane, Retin-A®, and tetracycline. However, use of these drugs is discouraged by pregnant women or women trying to conceive and should be thoroughly discussed with your health care provider and dermatologist.

What are these drugs?

Accutane: Accutane is a prescription medication that is taken orally to treat acne. The generic name for Accutane is isotretinoin.

Retina-A: Retin-A is a prescription cream that is applied to the skin to treat acne. The generic name for Retin-A is tretinoin.

Tetracycline: Tetracycline is an antibiotic taken orally to treat acne and respiratory infections.

What are the precautions?

Accutane (Category X): According to the Organization of Teratology Information Services (OTIS), approximately 25–35% of infants born to women exposed to Accutane during the first trimester of pregnancy showed a pattern of birth defects. This pattern includes craniofacial defects, heart defects, and central nervous system defects. There also is an increased risk of miscarriage and infant death associated with use of Accutane during pregnancy.

Retin-A (Category C): According to OTIS, less than 10% of Retin-A passes into the mother's blood stream and less than that reaches the baby. Even with these findings, Retin-A still carries warnings of use by women who are pregnant or contemplating pregnancy. In this case, it is best to discuss treatment with your dermatologist and other health care providers.

Tetracycline (Category D): According to OTIS, tetracycline appears to cause some inhibition of bone growth and discoloration of teeth in a fetus. Therefore, taking tetracycline should also be discussed with your dermatologist and other health care providers.

When is it safe to use these drugs?

Accutane: It is safe to use Accutane when you are not pregnant and have discussed certain guidelines with your health care provider.

- If you are in your childbearing years, you must use two forms of birth control, beginning one month prior to starting Accutane through one month after stopping Accutane. If you are breastfeeding, you should not take Accutane.

- You must be counseled about the possible ways that your chosen birth control may fail.

- You must have a negative pregnancy test one week prior to taking Accutane.

- You must start Accutane on the second or third day after the next normal menstrual period.

Retin-A: Since not many studies have been done on Retin-A, it is best to avoid during pregnancy and follow the same guidelines as Accutane while consulting with your health care provider.

Tetracycline: Tetracycline should not be used during pregnancy unless recommended by your health care provider. The American Academy of Pediatrics has approved tetracycline safe for use during breastfeeding.

What about over-the-counter acne medicated creams and astringents?

When choosing over-the-counter medicated acne cleansers and treatments, it is advised that you consult with your health care provider first. There are products that contain benzoyl peroxide, which have been recommended safe for pregnant women to use. However, there are over-the-counter medications that you may want to avoid such as products containing salicylic acids. Always consult your health care provider before taking any medications during pregnancy, whether prescription or over-the-counter.

Also, keep in mind that other things like caffeine, vitamins, herbal remedies, supplements, and herbal teas and remedies can affect the growing fetus. Talk with your health care provider about cutting down on caffeine and the type of vitamins you need to take. Never use any herbal product without talking to your health care provider first.

What over-the-counter and prescription drugs are not safe to take during pregnancy?

The Food and Drug Administration (FDA) has a system to rate drugs in terms of their safety during pregnancy. This system rates both over-the-counter (OTC) drugs you can buy in a drug or discount store and drugs your health care provider prescribes, but most medicines have not been studied in pregnant women to see if they cause damage to the growing fetus. Always talk with your health care provider if you have questions or concerns.

The FDA system ranks drugs as follows:

- **Category A:** Drugs that have been tested for safety during pregnancy and have been found to be safe. This includes drugs such as folic acid, vitamin B6, and thyroid medicine in moderation or in prescribed doses.

- **Category B:** Drugs that have been used a lot during pregnancy and do not appear to cause major birth defects or other problems. This includes drugs such as some antibiotics, acetaminophen (Tylenol®), aspartame (artificial sweetener), famotidine (Pepcid®), prednisone (cortisone), insulin (for diabetes), and ibuprofen (Advil®, Motrin®) before the third trimester. Pregnant women should not take ibuprofen during the last three months of pregnancy.

- **Category C:** Drugs that are more likely to cause problems for the mother or fetus. Also includes drugs for which safety studies have not been finished. The majority of these drugs do not have safety studies in progress. These drugs often come with a warning that they should be used only if the benefits of taking them outweigh the risks. This is something a woman would need to carefully discuss with her doctor. These drugs include prochlorperazine (Compazine®), Sudafed®, fluconazole (Diflucan®), and ciprofloxacin (Cipro®). Some antidepressants are also included in this group.

- **Category D:** Drugs that have clear health risks for the fetus and include alcohol, lithium (used to treat manic depression), phenytoin (Dilantin®), and most chemotherapy drugs to treat cancer. While these drugs are generally best avoided in pregnancy, there are some situations where their benefits to the mother will outweigh the risks to the fetus. For example, in some cases, chemotherapy drugs are given during pregnancy.

- **Category X:** Drugs that have been shown to cause birth defects and should never be taken during pregnancy. This includes drugs to treat skin conditions like cystic acne (Accutane®) and psoriasis (Tegison® or Soriatane®); a sedative (thalidomide); and a drug to prevent miscarriage used up until 1971 in the United States and 1983 in Europe (diethylstilbestrol or DES).

Aspirin and other drugs containing salicylate are not recommended during pregnancy, especially during the last three months. In rare cases, a woman's health care provider may want her to use these types of drugs under close watch. Acetylsalicylate, a common ingredient in many OTC painkillers, may make a pregnancy last longer and may cause severe bleeding before and after delivery.

Will there be studies in the future that will look at whether certain medicines or products are safe in pregnant women?

To help women make informed and educated decisions about using medicines during pregnancy, it is necessary to find out the effect of these medicines on the unborn baby. Pregnancy Registries are one way to do this. A Pregnancy Registry is a study that enrolls pregnant women after they have been taking medicine and before the birth of the baby. Babies born to women taking a particular medicine are compared with babies of women not taking the medicine. Looking at a large number of women and babies is needed to find out the effect of the medicine on the babies.

Should I avoid taking any medicine while I am pregnant?

Whether or not you should continue taking medicine during pregnancy is a serious question; but if you stop taking medicine that you need, this could harm both you and your baby. An example of this is if you have an infection called toxoplasmosis, which you can get from handling cat feces or eating infected meat. It can cause problems with the brain, eyes, heart, and other organs of a growing fetus. This infection requires treatment with antibiotics.

For pregnant women living with HIV, the Centers for Disease Control and Prevention (CDC) recommends antiretroviral drug therapy. Studies have found that HIV positive women who take antiviral drugs during pregnancy decrease by two-thirds the risk of passing HIV to their babies. If a diabetic woman does not take her medicine during pregnancy, she increases her risk for miscarriage and stillbirth. If asthma and/or high blood pressure are not controlled during pregnancy, problems with the fetus may result. Talk with your health care provider about whether the benefits of taking a medication outweigh the risk for you and your baby.

What about taking natural medications, or herbal remedies, when you are pregnant?

While some herbal remedies say they will help with pregnancy, there have been no studies to figure out if these claims are true. Likewise, there have been very few studies to look at how safe and effective herbal remedies are. Echinacea, ginkgo biloba, and St. John's wort have been popular herbs, to name a few, but there is little known about how they affect developing fetuses. It is probably safest to avoid herbal products entirely during pregnancy. Certainly, do not take any herbal products without talking to your health care provider first. These products may contain agents that could harm you and the growing fetus and cause problems with your pregnancy.

Chapter 20

X-Rays During Pregnancy

Pregnancy is a time to take good care of yourself and your unborn child. Many things are especially important during pregnancy, such as eating right, cutting out cigarettes and alcohol, and being careful about the prescription and over-the-counter drugs you take. Diagnostic x-rays and other medical radiation procedures of the abdominal area also deserve extra attention during pregnancy.

Diagnostic x-rays can give the doctor important, and even life-saving information, about a person's medical condition; but like many things, diagnostic x-rays have risks as well as benefits. They should be used only when they will give the doctor information needed to treat you.

You will probably never need an abdominal x-ray during pregnancy; but sometimes, because of a particular medical condition, your physician may feel that a diagnostic x-ray of your abdomen or lower torso is needed. If this should happen, do not be upset. The risk to you and your unborn child is very small, and the benefit of finding out about your medical condition is far greater.

You can reduce those risks by telling your doctor if you are, or think you might be, pregnant whenever an abdominal x-ray is prescribed. If you are

About This Chapter: Information in this chapter is from "X-Rays, Pregnancy and You," Center for Devices and Radiological Health, U.S. Food and Drug Administration (FDA), HHS Publication No. (FDA) 94-8087, May 2001. Reviewed December 2006 by David A. Cooke, M.D., Diplomate, American Board of Internal Medicine.

pregnant, the doctor may decide that it would be best to cancel the x-ray examination, to postpone it, or to modify it to reduce the amount of radiation; or, depending on your medical needs, and realizing that the risk is very small, the doctor may feel that it is best to proceed with the x-ray as planned. In any case, you should feel free to discuss the decision with your doctor.

✤ It's A Fact!!
The risk of not having a needed x-ray could be much greater than the risk from the radiation; but even small risks should not be taken if they are unnecessary.

What kind of x-rays can affect my unborn child?

During most x-ray examinations, like those of the arms, legs, head, teeth, or chest, your reproductive organs are not exposed to the direct x-ray beam. These kinds of procedures, when properly done, do not involve any risk to the unborn child. However, x-rays of the mother's lower torso, abdomen, stomach, pelvis, lower back, or kidneys, may expose the unborn child to the direct x-ray beam. They are of more concern.

What are the possible effects of x-rays?

There is scientific disagreement about whether the small amounts of radiation used in diagnostic radiology can actually harm the unborn child, but it is known that the unborn child is very sensitive to the effects of things like radiation, certain drugs, excess alcohol, and infection. This is true, in part, because the cells are rapidly dividing and growing into specialized cells and tissues. If radiation or other agents were to cause changes in these cells, there could be a slightly increased chance of birth defects or certain illnesses, such as leukemia, later in life.

It should be pointed out, however, that the majority of birth defects and childhood diseases occur even if the mother is not exposed to any known harmful agent during pregnancy. Scientists believe that heredity and random errors in the developmental process are responsible for most of these problems.

What if I'm x-rayed before I know I'm pregnant?

Do not be alarmed. Remember that the possibility of any harm to you and your unborn child from an x-ray is very small. There are, however, rare situations in which a woman who is unaware of her pregnancy may receive a very large number of abdominal x-rays over a short period; or she may receive radiation treatment of the lower torso. Under these circumstances, the woman should discuss the possible risks with her doctor.

How can I help minimize the risks?

To minimize the risks, you should do the following:

- Most important, tell your physician if you are pregnant or think you might be. This is important for many medical decisions, such as drug prescriptions and nuclear medicine procedures, as well as x-rays. And remember, this is true even in the very early weeks of pregnancy.

- Occasionally, a woman may mistake the symptoms of pregnancy for the symptoms of a disease. If you have any of the symptoms of pregnancy such as nausea, vomiting, breast tenderness, or fatigue, consider whether you might be pregnant and tell your doctor or x-ray technologist (the person doing the examination) before having an x-ray of the lower torso. A pregnancy test may be called for.

- If you are pregnant, or think you might be, do not hold a child who is being x-rayed. If you are not pregnant and you are asked to hold a child during an x-ray, be sure to ask for a lead apron to protect your reproductive organs. This is to prevent damage to your genes that could be passed on and cause harmful effects in your future descendants.

- Whenever an x-ray is requested, tell your doctor about any similar x-rays you have had recently. It may not be necessary to do another. It is a good idea to keep a record of the x-ray examinations you and your family have had taken so you can provide this kind of information accurately.

- Feel free to talk with your doctor about the need for an x-ray examination. You should understand the reason x-rays are requested in your particular case.

Chapter 21

Caffeine Use During Pregnancy

Caffeine is one of the most loved stimulants in America; but now that you are pregnant, you may need to lighten up on the daily intake of your favorite drinks and treats.

Facts About Caffeine

Caffeine is a stimulant and a diuretic. Because caffeine is a stimulant, it increases your blood pressure and heart rate, both of which are not recommended during pregnancy. Caffeine also increases the frequency of urination. This causes reduction in your body fluid levels and can lead to dehydration.

Caffeine crosses the placenta to your baby. Although you may be able to handle the amounts of caffeine you feed your body, your baby cannot. Your baby's metabolism is still maturing and cannot fully metabolize the caffeine. Any amount of caffeine can also cause changes in your baby's sleep pattern or normal movement pattern in the later stages of pregnancy.

Caffeine is found in more than just coffee. Caffeine is not only found in coffee but also in tea, soda, chocolate, and even some over-the-counter medications that relieve headaches. Be aware of what you consume.

About This Chapter: Information in this chapter is from "What's the Real Scoop on Caffeine During Pregnancy." Reprinted with permission from the American Pregnancy Association, http://www.americanpregnancy.org, © 2006. All rights reserved.

Fact Or Myth?

Caffeine causes birth defects. Numerous studies on animals have shown that caffeine can cause birth defects, preterm delivery, reduced fertility, and increase the risk of low-birth weight offspring, and other reproductive problems. There have not been any conclusive studies done on humans, though. It is still better to play it safe when it comes to inconclusive studies.

Caffeine causes infertility. Some studies have shown a link between high levels of caffeine consumption and delayed conception.

Caffeine causes miscarriages. A few studies have shown that there may be an increase in miscarriages among women who consume more than 300 mg (three 5 oz cups of coffee) a day. Other outcomes include preterm labor and low-birth weight babies. Again, it is safer to avoid caffeine as much as possible.

A pregnant woman should not consume any caffeine. Experts and studies have stated that "moderate" levels of caffeine have not been found to have a negative effect on pregnancy. The definition of "moderate" varies anywhere from 150 mg to 300 mg a day.

How Much Caffeine Is In Your Favorite Drinks And Snacks?

- Starbucks Grande Coffee (16 oz) 400 mg
- Starbucks House Blend Coffee (16 oz) 259 mg
- Dr. Pepper (12 oz) 37 mg
- 7 Eleven Big Gulp Diet Coke (32 oz) 124 mg
- 7 Eleven Big Gulp Coca-Cola (32 oz) 92 mg
- Ben and Jerry's Coffee Buzz Ice Cream (8 oz) 72 mg
- Baker's chocolate (1 oz) 26 mg
- Green tea (6 oz) 40 mg
- Black tea (8 oz) 60 mg

☞ **Remember!!**

Caffeine is a stimulant and can keep both you and your baby awake.

How Much Caffeine Is Too Much?

The less caffeine you consume, the better. Some experts say more than 150 mg of caffeine a day is too much, while others say more than 300 mg a day is too much. Avoiding caffeine as much as possible is your safest course of action. If you must get your fix, it is best to discuss this with your health care provider to make the healthiest choice for you and your baby.

Chapter 22

Smoking During Pregnancy

In the United States, more than 20 percent of women smoke. According to the World Health Organization, a similar number of women in other developed countries smoke, and about 9 percent of women in developing countries smoke. Many of these women smoke while they are pregnant. This is a major public health problem because, not only can smoking harm a woman's health, but smoking during pregnancy can lead to pregnancy complications and serious health problems in newborns.

Cigarette smoke contains more than 2,500 chemicals. It is not known for certain which of these chemicals are harmful to a developing baby. However, both nicotine and carbon monoxide are believed to play a role in causing adverse pregnancy outcomes.

How can smoke harm the newborn?

Smoking nearly doubles a woman's risk of having a low birth weight baby. In 2002, 12.2 percent of babies born to smokers in the United States were of low birth weight (less than 5½ pounds) compared to 7.5 percent of babies of nonsmokers. Low birth weight can result from poor growth before birth, preterm delivery, or a combination of both. Smoking has long been known to slow fetal growth. Studies also suggest that smoking increases the risk of preterm delivery (37 weeks of gestation). Premature and low birth weight babies face an increased risk of serious health problems during the newborn period, chronic lifelong disabilities (such as cerebral palsy, mental retardation, and learning problems), and even death.

The more a pregnant woman smokes, the greater the risk to her baby. However, if a woman stops smoking by the end of her first trimester of pregnancy, she is no more likely to have a low birth weight baby than a woman who never smoked. Even if a woman has not been able to stop smoking in her first or second trimester, stopping during the third trimester can still improve her baby's growth.

> **♣ It's A Fact!!**
>
> Statistics from the United States are compelling. If all pregnant women in the United States stopped smoking, there would be an estimated 11 percent reduction in stillbirths and a 5 percent reduction in newborn deaths, according to the U.S. Public Health Service. Currently, at least 11 percent of women in the United States smoke during pregnancy.

Can smoking cause pregnancy complications?

Smoking has been associated with a number of pregnancy complications. Smoking cigarettes appears to double a woman's risk of developing placental problems. These include placenta previa (low-lying placenta that covers part or all of the opening of the uterus) and placental abruption (in which the placenta peels away, partially or almost completely, from the uterine wall before delivery). Both can result in heavy bleeding during delivery that can endanger mother and baby, although a cesarean delivery can prevent most deaths. Placental problems contribute to the slightly increased risk of stillbirth that is associated with smoking.

Smoking in pregnancy also appears to increase a woman's risk of premature rupture of the membranes (PROM) (when the sac inside the uterus that holds the baby breaks before labor begins). A woman with PROM may experience a trickle or gush of fluid from her vagina when her water breaks. Usually, she will go into labor within a few hours. When PROM occurs before 37 weeks of pregnancy, it is called preterm PROM, and it often results in the birth of a premature baby.

Does smoking affect fertility?

Cigarette smoking can cause reproductive problems before a woman even becomes pregnant. Studies show that women who smoke may have more trouble conceiving than nonsmokers. Studies suggest that fertility returns to normal after a woman stops smoking.

Does smoking during pregnancy cause other problems in babies or young children?

A recent study suggests that babies of mothers who smoke during pregnancy may undergo withdrawal-like symptoms similar to those seen in babies of mothers who use some illicit drugs. For example, babies of smokers appear to be more jittery and difficult to soothe than babies of non-smokers.

Babies whose mothers smoked during pregnancy are up to three times as likely to die from sudden infant death syndrome (SIDS) as babies of non-smokers.

Can exposure to secondhand smoke during pregnancy harm the baby?

Studies suggest that babies of women who are regularly exposed to secondhand smoke during pregnancy may have reduced growth and may be more likely to be born with low birth weight. Pregnant women who do not smoke should avoid exposure to other people's smoke.

How can a woman stop smoking?

The March of Dimes recommends that women stop smoking before they become pregnant and remain smoke-free throughout pregnancy and after the baby is born. A woman's health care provider can refer her to a smoking cessation program that is right for her or suggest other ways to help her quit. The March of Dimes supports a 5- to 15-minute, 5-step counseling approach called "The 5 A's," which is performed by the health care provider during routine prenatal visits. This approach has been shown to improve smoking cessation rates by 30 to 70 percent among pregnant women. Even later in pregnancy, a woman can reduce the risks to her baby by stopping smoking.

Studies suggest that certain factors make it more likely that a woman will be successful in her efforts to quit smoking during pregnancy. These include attempting to quit in the past, having a partner who does not smoke, getting support from family or other important people in her life, and understanding the harmful effects of smoking.

How does exposure to smoke after birth affect a baby?

It is important to stay smoke-free after the baby is born. Both mother and father should refrain from smoking in the home and should ask visitors to do the same. Babies who are exposed to smoke suffer from more lower respiratory illnesses (such as bronchitis and pneumonia) and ear infections than other babies. Babies who are exposed to their parents' smoke after birth also may face an increased risk of SIDS. A child exposed to smoking at home during the first few years of life also is at increased risk of developing asthma.

Of course, smoking harms a woman's own health. Smokers have an increased risk of lung and other cancers, heart disease, stroke, and emphysema (a potentially disabling and, sometimes, deadly lung condition). Quitting smoking will make parents healthier and better role models for their children.

Chapter 23

Alcohol Consumption During Pregnancy

What are FAS and FASDs?

Prenatal exposure to alcohol can cause a range of disorders, known as fetal alcohol spectrum disorders (FASDs). One of the most severe effects of drinking during pregnancy is fetal alcohol syndrome (FAS). FAS is one of the leading known preventable causes of mental retardation and birth defects. If a woman drinks alcohol during her pregnancy, her baby can be born with FAS, a lifelong condition that causes physical and mental disabilities. FAS is characterized by abnormal facial features, growth deficiencies, and central nervous system (CNS) problems. People with FAS might have problems with learning, memory, attention span, communication, vision, hearing, or a combination of these. These problems often lead to difficulties in school and problems getting along with others. FAS is a permanent condition. It affects every aspect of an individual's life and the lives of his or her family.

FASDs include FAS, as well as other conditions, in which individuals have some, but not all, of the clinical signs of FAS. Three terms often used are fetal alcohol effects (FAE), alcohol-related neurodevelopmental disorder (ARND), and alcohol-related birth defects (ARBD). The term FAE has been used to describe behavioral and cognitive problems in children who were prenatally

About This Chapter: Information in this chapter is from "Fetal Alcohol Spectrum Disorders," National Center on Birth Defects and Developmental Disabilities, Centers for Disease Control and Prevention (CDC), May 2006.

exposed to alcohol, but who do not have all of the typical diagnostic features of FAS. In 1996, the Institute of Medicine (IOM) replaced FAE with the terms ARND and ARBD. Children with ARND might have functional or mental problems linked to prenatal alcohol exposure. These include behavioral or cognitive abnormalities or a combination of both. Children with ARBD might have problems with the heart, kidneys, bones, and/or hearing.

All FASDs are 100% preventable if a woman does not drink alcohol while she is pregnant.

How common are FAS and FASDs?

The reported rates of FAS vary widely. These different rates depend on the population studied and the surveillance methods used. Centers for Disease Control and Prevention (CDC) studies show FAS rates ranging from 0.2 to 1.5 per 1,000 live births in different areas of the United States. Other FASDs are believed to occur approximately three times as often as FAS.

What are the characteristics of children with FAS and other FASDs?

FAS is the severe end of a spectrum of effects that can occur when a woman drinks during pregnancy. Fetal death is the most extreme outcome. FAS is a disorder characterized by abnormal facial features and growth and central nervous system (CNS) problems. If a pregnant woman drinks alcohol, but her child does not have all of the symptoms of FAS, it is possible that her child has another FASD, such as alcohol-related neurodevelopmental disorder (ARND). Children with ARND do not have full FAS but might demonstrate learning and behavioral problems caused by prenatal exposure to alcohol. Examples of these problems are difficulties with mathematical skills, difficulties with memory or attention, poor school performance, and poor impulse control and/or judgment.

Children with FASDs might have the following characteristics or exhibit the following behaviors:

- small size for gestational age or small stature in relation to peers

- facial abnormalities such as small eye openings

- poor coordination

> ## ♣ It's A Fact!!
>
> Fetal alcohol spectrum disorders (FASDs) is an umbrella term describing the range of effects that can occur in an individual whose mother drank alcohol during pregnancy. These effects include physical, mental, behavioral, and/or learning disabilities with possible lifelong implications. The term FASDs is not intended for use as a clinical diagnosis.

- hyperactive behavior
- learning disabilities
- developmental disabilities (e.g., speech and language delays)
- mental retardation or low IQ
- problems with daily living
- poor reasoning and judgment skills
- sleep and sucking disturbances in infancy

Children with FASDs are at risk for psychiatric problems, criminal behavior, unemployment, and incomplete education. These are secondary conditions that an individual is not born with but might acquire as a result of FAS or a related disorder. These conditions can be very serious, but there are protective factors that have been found to help individuals with FASDs. For example, a child who is diagnosed early in life can be placed in appropriate educational classes and given access to social services that can help the child and his or her family. Children with FASDs who receive special education are more likely to achieve their developmental and educational potential. In addition, children with FASDs need a loving, nurturing, and stable home life to avoid disruptions, transient lifestyles, or harmful relationships. Children with FASDs who live in abusive or unstable homes, or who become involved in youth violence, are much more likely than those who do not have such negative experiences to develop secondary conditions.

How can we prevent FASDs?

FASDs are completely preventable if a woman does not drink alcohol while she is pregnant or could become pregnant. If a woman is drinking during pregnancy, it is never too late for her to stop. The sooner a woman stops drinking, the better it will be for both her baby and herself. If a woman is not able to stop drinking, she should contact her doctor, local Alcoholics Anonymous, or local alcohol treatment center. The Substance Abuse and

Mental Health Services Administration has a Substance Abuse Treatment Facility locator. This locator helps people find drug and alcohol treatment programs in their area. If a woman is sexually active and is not using an effective form of birth control, she should not drink alcohol. She could become pregnant and not know it for several weeks or more.

Chapter 24

Illegal Drug Use During Pregnancy

When you are pregnant it is important that you watch what you put into your body. Consumption of illegal drugs is not safe for the unborn baby or for the mother.

The following information can help you understand these drugs and their effects.

Marijuana

What are the common slang names?

The common slang names are pot, weed, grass, and reefer.

What happens when a pregnant woman smokes marijuana?

Marijuana crosses the placenta to your baby. Marijuana, like cigarette smoke, contains toxins that keep your baby from getting the proper supply of oxygen that he or she needs to grow.

How can marijuana affect the unborn baby?

Studies of marijuana in pregnancy are inconclusive because many women who smoke marijuana also use tobacco and alcohol. Smoking marijuana

About This Chapter: Information in this chapter is from "Using Illegal Street Drugs During Pregnancy." Reprinted with permission from the American Pregnancy Association, http://www.americanpregnancy.org, © 2006. All rights reserved.

increases the levels of carbon monoxide and carbon dioxide in the blood, which reduces the oxygen supply to the baby. Smoking marijuana during pregnancy can increase the chance of miscarriage, low birth weight, premature birth, developmental delays, and behavioral and learning problems.

♣ It's A Fact!!

Studies have shown that consumption of illegal drugs during pregnancy can result in miscarriage, low birth weight, premature labor, placental abruption, fetal death, and even maternal death.

What if I smoked marijuana before I knew I was pregnant?

According to Dr. Richard S. Abram, author of *Will it Hurt the Baby*, "occasional use of marijuana during the first trimester is unlikely to cause birth defects." Once you are aware you are pregnant, you should stop smoking. Doing this will decrease the chance of harming your baby.

Cocaine

What are the common slang names?

The common slang names are bump, toot, C, coke, crack, flake, snow, and candy.

What happens when a pregnant woman consumes cocaine?

Cocaine crosses the placenta and enters your baby's circulation. The elimination of cocaine is slower in a fetus than in an adult. This means that cocaine remains in the baby's body much longer than it does in your body.

How can cocaine affect my unborn baby?

According to the Organization of Teratology Information Services (OTIS), during the early months of pregnancy cocaine exposure may increase the risk of miscarriage. Later in pregnancy, cocaine use can cause placental abruption. Placental abruption can lead to severe bleeding, preterm birth, and fetal death. OTIS also states that the risk of a birth defect appears to be greater when the mother has used cocaine frequently during pregnancy.

According to the American College of Obstetricians and Gynecology (ACOG), women who use cocaine during their pregnancy have a 25% increased chance of premature labor. Babies born to mothers who use cocaine throughout their pregnancy may also have a smaller head and their growth hindered. Babies who are exposed to cocaine later in pregnancy may be born dependent and suffer from withdrawal symptoms such as tremors, sleeplessness, muscle spasms, and difficulties feeding. Some experts believe that learning difficulties may result as the child gets older. Defects of the genitals, kidneys, and brain are also possible.

What if I consumed cocaine before I knew I was pregnant?

There have not been any conclusive studies done on single doses of cocaine during pregnancy. Birth defects and other side effects are usually a result of prolonged use; but because studies are inconclusive, it is best to avoid cocaine altogether. Cocaine is a very addictive drug, and experimentation often leads to abuse of the drug.

Heroin

What are the common slang names?

The common slang names are horse, smack, junk, and H-stuff.

What happens when a pregnant woman uses heroin?

Heroin is a very addictive drug that crosses the placenta to the baby. Because this drug is so addictive, the unborn baby can become dependent on the drug.

How can heroin affect my unborn baby?

Using heroin during pregnancy increases the chance of premature birth, low birth weight, breathing difficulties, low blood sugar (hypoglycemia), bleeding within the brain (intracranial hemorrhage), and infant death. Babies can also be born addicted to heroin and can suffer from withdrawal symptoms. Withdrawal symptoms include irritability, convulsions, diarrhea, fever, sleep abnormalities, and joint stiffness. Mothers who inject narcotics are more susceptible to HIV, which can be passed to their unborn child.

What if I am addicted to heroin, and I am pregnant?

Treating an addiction to heroin can be complicated, especially when you are pregnant. Your health care provider may prescribe methadone as a form of treatment. It is best that you communicate with your health care provider so he or she can provide the best treatment for you and your baby.

PCP And LSD

What happens when a pregnant woman takes PCP and LSD?

PCP and LSD are hallucinogens. Both PCP and LSD users can have violent behavior, which may cause harm to the baby if the mother hurts herself.

How can PCP and LSD affect my unborn baby?

PCP use during pregnancy can lead to low birth weight, poor muscle control, brain damage, and withdrawal syndrome if used frequently. Withdrawal symptoms include lethargy, alternating with tremors. LSD can lead to birth defects if used frequently.

What if I experimented with LSD or PCP before I knew I was pregnant?

No conclusive studies have been done on one-time use effects of these drugs on the fetus. It is best not to experiment if you think you might be pregnant.

Methamphetamine

What are the common slang names?

The common slang names are meth, speed, crystal, glass, and crank.

What happens when a pregnant woman takes methamphetamine?

Methamphetamine is chemically related to amphetamine, which causes the heart rate of the mother and baby to increase.

How can methamphetamine affect my unborn baby?

Taking methamphetamine during pregnancy can result in problems similar to those seen with the use of cocaine in pregnancy. The use of speed can cause the baby to get less oxygen, which can lead to a small baby at birth. Methamphetamine can also increase the likelihood of premature labor, miscarriage, and placental abruption. Babies can be born addicted to methamphetamine and suffer withdrawal symptoms that include tremors, sleeplessness, muscle spasms, and difficulties feeding. Some experts believe that learning difficulties may result as the child gets older.

What if I experimented with methamphetamine before I knew I was pregnant?

There have not been any significant studies done on the effect of one time use of methamphetamine during pregnancy. It is best not to experiment if you think you might be pregnant.

What Does The Law Say?

Currently there is only one state, South Carolina, who holds prenatal substance abuse as a criminal act of child abuse and neglect. Other states have laws that address prenatal substance abuse:

- Iowa, Minnesota, and North Dakota's health care providers are required to report and test for prenatal drug exposure. Virginia health care providers are only required to test.

- Arizona, Illinois, Massachusetts, Michigan, Utah, and Rhode Island's health care providers are required to report prenatal drug exposure. Reporting and testing can be evidence used in child welfare proceedings.

- Some states consider prenatal substance abuse as part of their child welfare laws. Therefore, prenatal drug exposure can provide grounds for terminating parental rights because of child abuse or neglect. These states include: Colorado, Florida, Illinois, Indiana, Maryland, Minnesota, Nevada, Ohio, Rhode Island, South Carolina, South Dakota, Texas, Virginia, and Wisconsin.

- Some states have policies that enforce admission to an inpatient treatment program for pregnant women who use drugs. These states include: Minnesota, South Dakota, and Wisconsin.

- In 2004, Texas made it a felony to smoke marijuana while pregnant, resulting in a prison sentence of 2–20 years.

✔ Quick Tip
How Can I Get Help?

You can get help from counseling, support groups, and treatment programs. Popular groups include the 12-step program. Numbers that can help you locate a treatment center include the following:

- National Drug Help Hotline 800-662-4357

- National Alcohol and Drug Dependence Hopeline 800-622-2255

Chapter 25

Environmental Risks And Pregnancy

There are more than four million chemical mixtures in homes and businesses in this country with little information on the effects of most of them during pregnancy. However, a few are known to be harmful to an unborn baby. Most of these are found in the workplace, but certain environmental pollutants found in air and water, as well as chemicals used at home, may pose a risk during pregnancy.

A pregnant woman can inhale these chemicals, ingest them in food or drink, or, in some cases, absorb them through the skin. For most hazardous substances, a pregnant woman would have to be exposed to a large amount for a long time in order for them to harm her baby. Most workplaces have preventive measures to help make sure this does not happen. Pregnant women can take steps to help protect themselves and their babies from pollutants and potentially risky chemicals used at home.

What are the risks of lead exposure during pregnancy?

Lead is a naturally occurring metal that was found for many years in gasoline, paint, and other products used in homes and businesses. While lead is still present in the environment, the amounts continue to decrease

since the Environmental Protection Agency
(EPA) banned its use in these products in
the 1970s.

♣ It's A Fact!!

Lead poses health risks for
everyone, but young children
and unborn babies are at
greatest risk.

Exposure to high levels of lead during pregnancy contributes to miscarriage,
preterm delivery, low birth weight, and developmental delays in the infant. Lead toxic-
ity in children is characterized by behavioral and
learning problems and anemia. Few pregnant women in the United States
are exposed to high levels of lead. However, even low levels of exposure may
cause subtle learning and behavioral problems in the child.

Women who live in older homes may be exposed to higher levels of lead
due to deteriorating lead-based paint. About 80 percent of homes built before
1978 were painted with lead-based paint. As long as paint is not crumbling or
peeling, it poses little risk. However, if lead-based paint needs to be removed
from a home, pregnant women and children should stay out of the home until
the project is complete. Sanding or scraping leaded paint produces lead dust.
Only experts should remove leaded paint using proper precautions.

Occasionally, a pregnant woman is exposed to significant amounts of lead in
her drinking water if her home has lead pipes, lead solder on copper pipes, or
brass faucets. Pregnant women can contact their state health department to find
out how to get their pipes tested for lead. The EPA recommends running water
for 30 seconds before using it for drinking or cooking to help reduce lead levels.
A pregnant woman should use only water from the cold water pipe, which contains less lead than hot water, for cooking, drinking, and preparing baby formula.
Many home filters do not remove lead, so a pregnant woman should read the
label on her filter carefully and change the filter as recommended.

Lead crystal glassware and some ceramic dishes may contain lead, and
pregnant women and children should avoid frequent use of these items.
Commercial ceramics are safer than those made by craftspeople. Other unexpected sources of lead in the home may include the wicks of scented candles
(which release lead particles into the air when burned) and the plastic (poly-
vinyl chloride) grips on some hand tools.

Some arts and crafts materials (e.g., oil paints, ceramic glazes, and stained glass materials) contain lead. A woman should try to stick with lead-free alternatives (such as acrylic or watercolor paints) during pregnancy and breastfeeding.

If anyone in the home is exposed to lead on the job (such as painters and those working in smelters, auto repair shops, battery manufacturing plants, or certain types of construction), they should change their clothing and shower at work to avoid bringing lead into the home. They should wash contaminated clothing at work, if possible, or wash it at home separately from the rest of the family's clothing.

Does mercury exposure pose a risk in pregnancy?

Mercury is another metal that is present naturally in the environment. Pregnant women are most often exposed to mercury by eating contaminated fish. Mercury enters the environment from natural and man-made sources (such as coal-burning or other industrial pollution). It is converted by bacteria to a more dangerous form (methyl mercury) that accumulates in the fatty tissues of fish. While trace amounts of mercury are present in many types of fish, mercury is most concentrated in large fish that eat other fish such as swordfish and sharks.

In 2004, the U.S. Food and Drug Administration (FDA) and the Environmental Protection Agency (EPA) made three recommendations for women who might become pregnant, women who are pregnant, and nursing mothers. By following these recommendations, women can get the benefits of eating fish and shellfish and be confident that they have reduced their exposure to the harmful effects of mercury.

1. Do not eat shark, swordfish, king mackerel, or tilefish because they contain high levels of mercury.

2. Eat up to 12 ounces (two average meals) a week of a variety of fish and shellfish that are lower in mercury. Five of the most commonly eaten fish that are low in mercury are shrimp, canned light tuna, salmon, pollock, and catfish. Another commonly eaten fish, albacore ("white") tuna, has more mercury than canned light tuna. When choosing two meals of fish and shellfish, women may eat up to 6 ounces (one average meal) of albacore tuna per week.

3. Check local advisories about the safety of fish caught by family and friends in local lakes, rivers, and coastal areas. If no advice is available, women may eat up to 6 ounces (one average meal) per week of fish caught from local waters, but they should not consume any other fish during that week.

Game fish also may be contaminated with other industrial pollutants such as PCBs (polychlorinated biphenyls). A pregnant woman's exposure to PCBs may contribute to a child's learning problems, reduced IQ, and low birth weight. Pregnant women or women who could become pregnant should not consume any game fish without checking with their state or local health department or the EPA to find out which fish are safe to eat.

It is less certain whether exposure to elemental mercury, which is used in thermometers, dental fillings, and batteries, poses a risk in pregnancy. Some studies have found an increased risk of miscarriage in women working in dental offices. Women who work with mercury should take all recommended precautions to reduce their exposure.

What other metals pose a risk in pregnancy?

Arsenic and cadmium are two other metals that are suspected of posing pregnancy risks. These metals enter the environment through natural (weathering of rock and forest fires) and man-made (mining and burning of fossil fuels and waste) forces.

While arsenic is a well-known poison, the small amounts normally found in the environment are unlikely to harm a fetus. However, certain women may be exposed to higher levels of arsenic that could pose a risk. Several studies suggest that women working at or living near metal smelters may be at increased risk of miscarriage and stillbirth. Women who live in agricultural areas where arsenic fertilizers (now banned) were used on crops or who live near hazardous waste sites or incinerators also may be exposed to higher-than-normal levels of arsenic. They can help protect themselves by having their water tested for arsenic or by drinking bottled water and limiting contact with soil. Because arsenic also is used as part of a preservative in pressure-treated lumber, pregnant women should avoid wood dust from home construction projects. Anyone who works with arsenic (semiconductor manufacturing, metal smelting, herbicide application) should avoid bringing the metal home on clothing.

Scientists suspect that cadmium may pose a risk in pregnancy. One study suggests that cadmium may damage the placenta and reduce birth weight. This metal is used in many occupations including semiconductor manufacturing, welding, soldering, ceramics, and painting. Women who work with cadmium should take all recommended precautions and avoid bringing it home on clothing. Pregnant women also may want to consider eliminating sources of cadmium from the house, such as fungicides containing cadmium chloride, certain fabric dyes, and ceramic and glass glazes and some fertilizers.

Can pesticides harm an unborn baby?

Pregnant women should avoid pesticides whenever possible. There is no proof that exposure to pest control products at levels commonly used at home pose a risk to the fetus. However, all insecticides are to some extent poisonous, and some studies have suggested that high levels of exposure to pesticides may contribute to miscarriage, preterm delivery, and birth defects. Certain pesticides and other chemicals, including PCBs, have weak, estrogen-like qualities called endocrine disrupters that some scientists suspect may affect development of the fetus's reproductive system.

♣ **It's A Fact!!**

Health care providers have some concerns about the use of insect repellants during pregnancy. The insect repellant DEET (diethyltoluamide) is among the most effective at keeping bugs from biting; however, its safety during pregnancy has not been fully assessed. If a pregnant woman uses DEET, she should not apply it to her skin. Instead, she should place small amounts on her socks and shoes and outer clothes using gloves or an applicator to avoid contact with her fingers.

A pregnant woman can reduce her exposure to pesticides by controlling pest problems with less toxic products such as boric acid (use the blue form available at hardware stores). If she must have her home or property treated with pesticides, a pregnant woman should do the following:

- Have someone else apply the chemicals and leave the area for the amount of time indicated on the package instructions.

- Remove food, dishes, and utensils from the area before the pesticide is applied. Afterwards, have someone open the windows and wash off all surfaces on which food is prepared.

- Close all windows and turn off air conditioning when pesticides are used outdoors, so fumes are not drawn into the house.

- Wear rubber gloves when gardening to prevent skin contact with pesticides.

What are organic solvents?

Organic solvents are chemicals that dissolve other substances. Common organic solvents include alcohols, degreasers, paint thinners, and varnish removers. Lacquers, silk-screening inks, and paints also contain these chemicals. A 1999 Canadian study found that women who were exposed to solvents on the job during their first trimester of pregnancy were about 13 times more likely than unexposed women to have a baby with a major birth defect, like spina bifida (open spine), clubfoot, heart defects, and deafness. The women in the study included factory workers, laboratory technicians, artists, graphic designers, and printing industry workers.

Other studies have found that women workers in semiconductor plants exposed to high levels of solvents, called glycol ethers, were almost three times more likely to miscarry than unexposed women. Glycol ethers also are used in jobs that involve photography, dyes, and silk-screen printing.

Pregnant women who work with solvents, including women who do arts and crafts at home, should minimize their exposure by making sure their workplace is well ventilated and by wearing appropriate protective equipment including gloves and a face mask. They should never eat or drink in their work area. To learn more about the chemicals she works with, a woman can ask her employer for the Material Safety Data Sheets for the products she uses or contact the National Institute for Occupational Safety and Health or visit http://www.msdssearch.com/.

Is drinking chlorinated tap water safe during pregnancy?

In recent years, media reports have raised concerns about possible pregnancy risks from by-products of chlorinated drinking water. Chlorine is added to drinking water to kill disease-causing microbes. However, when chlorine combines with other materials in water, it forms chloroform and related chemicals called trihalomethanes. The level of these chemicals in water supplies varies. A few studies suggest that the risk of miscarriage and poor fetal growth may be increased when levels of these chemicals are high, while other studies have not found an increased risk. Scientists continue to study the safety of these chemicals during pregnancy. Until we know more, pregnant women who are concerned about chlorine may choose to drink bottled water.

Drinking water also can become contaminated with pesticides, lead, or other metals. Women who suspect their water supply may be affected can have their water tested or drink bottled water.

Do household cleaning products pose a risk in pregnancy?

✔ Quick Tip

A pregnant woman who is worried about commercial cleansers or bothered by their odors can substitute safe, natural products. For example, baking soda can be used as a powdered cleanser to scrub greasy areas, pots and pans, sinks, tubs, and ovens. A solution of vinegar and water can effectively clean many surfaces such as countertops.

While some household cleansers contain solvents, there are many safe alternatives. Pregnant women should read labels carefully and avoid products (such as some oven cleaners) whose labels indicate they are toxic.

Products that contain ammonia or chlorine are unlikely to harm an unborn baby, though their odors may trigger nausea in a pregnant woman. A pregnant woman should open windows and doors and wear rubber gloves when using these products. She should never mix ammonia and chlorine products because the combination produces fumes that are dangerous for anyone.

Part Four

High-Risk Pregnancies
And Pregnancy Complications

Chapter 26

Risk Factors Present Before Pregnancy

Some risk factors are present before women become pregnant. These risk factors include certain physical and social characteristics of women, problems that have occurred in previous pregnancies, and certain disorders women already have.

Physical Characteristics

The age, weight, and height of women affect risk during pregnancy.

Women aged 35 and older are at increased risk of problems such as high blood pressure, gestational diabetes (diabetes that develops during pregnancy), and complications during labor.

Women who weigh less than 100 pounds before becoming pregnant are more likely to have small, underweight babies. Obese women are more likely to have very large babies, which may be difficult to deliver. Also, obese women are more likely to develop gestational diabetes and preeclampsia.

Women shorter than 5 feet are more likely to have a small pelvis, which may make movement of the fetus through the pelvis and vagina (birth canal) difficult

About This Chapter: Information in this chapter is from "Risk Factors Present Before Pregnancy," *The Merck Manual of Medical Information—Second Home Edition*, pp. 1444–1449, edited by Mark H. Beers. Copyright 2003 by Merck and Co., Inc., Whitehouse Station, NJ. Reprinted with permission. Merck Manuals are available free online at www.MerckManuals.com.

during labor. For example, the fetus's shoulder is more likely to lodge against the pubic bone. This complication is called shoulder dystocia. Also, short women are more likely to have preterm labor and a baby who has not grown as much as expected.

♣ It's A Fact!!
Girls aged 15 and younger are at increased risk of preeclampsia (a type of high blood pressure that develops during pregnancy). Young girls are also at increased risk of having underweight (small-for-gestational-age) or undernourished babies.

Structural abnormalities in the reproductive organs increase the risk of a miscarriage. Examples are a double uterus or a weak (incompetent) cervix that tends to open (dilate) as the fetus grows.

Social Characteristics

Being unmarried or in a lower socioeconomic group increases the risk of problems during pregnancy. The reason these characteristics increase risk is unclear but is probably related to other characteristics that are more common among these women. For example, these women are more likely to smoke and less likely to consume a healthy diet and to obtain appropriate medical care.

Problems In A Previous Pregnancy

When women have had a problem in one pregnancy, they are more likely to have a problem, often the same one, in subsequent pregnancies. Such problems include having had a premature baby, an underweight baby, a baby that weighed more than 10 pounds, a baby with birth defects, a previous miscarriage, a late (post term) delivery (after 42 weeks of pregnancy), Rh incompatibility that required a blood transfusion to the fetus, or a delivery that required a cesarean section. If women have had a baby who died shortly after birth, they are also more likely to have problems in subsequent pregnancies.

Women may have a condition that tends to make the same problem recur. For example, women with diabetes are more likely to have babies that weigh more than 10 pounds at birth.

Women who had a baby with a genetic disorder or birth defect are more likely to have another baby with a similar problem. Genetic testing of the baby, even if stillborn, and of both parents may be appropriate before another pregnancy is attempted. If these women become pregnant again, tests such as ultrasonography, chorionic villus sampling, and amniocentesis may help determine whether the fetus has a genetic disorder or birth defect.

Having had six or more pregnancies increases the risks of very rapid labor and excessive bleeding after delivery. It also increases the risk of a mislocated placenta (placenta previa).

Disorders Present Before Pregnancy

Before becoming pregnant, women may have a disorder that can increase the risk of problems during pregnancy. These women should talk with a doctor and try to get in the best physical condition possible before they become pregnant. After they become pregnant, they may need special care, often from an interdisciplinary team. The team may include an obstetrician (who may also be a specialist in the disorder), a specialist in the disorder, and other health care practitioners (such as nutritionists).

Heart Disease: Most women who have heart disease, including heart valve disorders (such as mitral valve prolapse) and some birth defects of the heart, can safely give birth to healthy children without any permanent ill effects on heart function or life span. However, women who have heart failure before pregnancy are at considerable risk of problems.

Pregnancy requires the heart to work harder. Consequently, pregnancy may worsen heart disease or cause heart disease to produce symptoms for the first time. Usually, serious problems, including death of the woman or fetus, occur only when heart disease is severe before the woman becomes pregnant. About 1% of women who have severe heart disease before becoming pregnant die as a result of the pregnancy, usually because of heart failure.

The risk of problems increases throughout pregnancy as demands on the heart increase. Pregnant women with heart disease may become unusually tired and may need to limit their activities. Rarely, women with severe heart disease are advised to have an abortion early in pregnancy. Risk is also increased during labor and delivery. After delivery, women with severe heart disease may not be out of danger for at least 6 months, depending on the type of heart disease.

Heart disease in pregnant women may affect the fetus. The fetus may be born prematurely. Women with birth defects of the heart are more likely to have children with similar birth defects. Ultrasonography can detect some of these defects before the fetus is born. If severe heart disease in a pregnant woman suddenly worsens, the fetus may die.

During labor, women who have severe heart disease may be given an epidural anesthetic, which blocks sensation in the lower spinal cord and prevents women from pushing. Pushing during labor strains the heart, because it increases the amount of blood returning to the heart. Because pushing is not possible, the baby may have to be delivered with forceps.

For women with some types of heart disease, pregnancy is inadvisable because it so increases their risk of death. Primary pulmonary hypertension and Eisenmenger syndrome are examples. If women who have one of these disorders become pregnant, doctors advise them to terminate the pregnancy as early as possible.

High Blood Pressure: Women who have high blood pressure (chronic hypertension) before they become pregnant are more likely to have potentially serious problems during pregnancy. These problems include preeclampsia (a type of high blood pressure that develops during pregnancy, worsening of high blood pressure, a fetus that does not grow as much as expected, premature detachment of the placenta from the uterus (placental abruption), and stillbirth.

For most women with moderately high blood pressure (140/90 to 150/100 millimeters of mercury [mm Hg]), treatment with antihypertensive drugs is not recommended. Such treatment does not seem to reduce the risk of preeclampsia, premature detachment of the placenta, or a stillbirth, or to improve the growth of the fetus. However, some women are treated to prevent pregnancy from causing episodes of even higher blood pressure, which require hospitalization.

For women whose blood pressure is higher than 150/100 mm Hg, treatment with antihypertensive drugs is recommended. Treatment can reduce the risk of stroke and other complications due to very high blood pressure. Treatment is also recommended for women who have high blood pressure and a kidney disorder, because if high blood pressure is not controlled well, the kidneys may be damaged further.

Most antihypertensive drugs used to treat high blood pressure can be used safely during pregnancy. However, angiotensin-converting enzyme (ACE) inhibitors are discontinued during pregnancy, particularly during the last two trimesters. These drugs can cause severe kidney damage in the fetus. As a result, the baby may die shortly after birth.

During pregnancy, women with high blood pressure are monitored closely to make sure blood pressure is well controlled, the kidneys are functioning normally, and the fetus is growing normally. However, premature detachment of the placenta cannot be prevented or anticipated. Often, a baby must be delivered early to prevent stillbirth or complications due to high blood pressure (such as stroke) in the woman.

Anemia: Having a hereditary anemia, such as sickle cell disease, hemoglobin S-C disease, and some thalassemias, increases the risk of problems during pregnancy. Before delivery, blood tests are routinely performed to check for hemoglobin abnormalities in women who are at increased risk of having these abnormalities because of race, ethnic background, or family history. Chorionic villus sampling or amniocentesis may be performed to detect a hemoglobin abnormality in the fetus.

Women who have sickle cell disease are particularly at risk of developing infections during pregnancy. Pneumonia, urinary tract infections, and infections of the uterus are the most common. About one third of pregnant women who have sickle cell disease develop high blood pressure during pregnancy. A sudden, severe attack of pain, called sickle cell crisis, may occur during pregnancy as at any other time. Heart failure and blockage of arteries of the lungs by blood clots (pulmonary embolism), which may be life threatening, may also occur. Bleeding during labor or after delivery may be more severe. The fetus may grow slowly or not as much as expected. The fetus may even die. The more severe sickle cell disease was before pregnancy, the higher the risk of health problems for pregnant women and the fetus and the higher the risk of death for the fetus during pregnancy. With regular blood transfusions, women are less likely to have sickle cell crises but are more likely to reject the transfused blood. This condition, called alloimmunization, can be life threatening. Also, transfusions to pregnant women do not reduce risks for the fetus.

Kidney Disorders: Women with a severe kidney disorder before pregnancy are more likely to have problems during pregnancy. Kidney function may rapidly worsen during pregnancy. High blood pressure, which often accompanies a kidney disorder, may also worsen, and preeclampsia (a type of high blood pressure that develops during pregnancy) may develop. The fetus may not grow as much as expected or may be stillborn. In pregnant women who have a kidney disorder, kidney function and blood pressure are monitored closely as is the growth of the fetus. Often, the baby must be delivered early.

Women who have had a kidney transplant that has been in place for two or more years are usually able to safely give birth to healthy babies if their kidneys are functioning normally, if they have had no episodes of rejection, and if their blood pressure is normal. Many women who have a kidney disorder and who undergo hemodialysis regularly can also give birth to healthy babies.

Seizure Disorders: For most women who take anticonvulsants to treat a seizure disorder, the frequency of seizures does not change during pregnancy. However, sometimes the dose of the anticonvulsant must be increased.

Taking anticonvulsants increases the risk of birth defects. Women who take anticonvulsants should discuss the risk of birth defects with an expert in the field, preferably before they become pregnant. Some women may be able to safely discontinue anticonvulsants during pregnancy, but most women should continue to take the drugs. The risks resulting from not taking the drugs (resulting in more frequent seizures, which can harm the fetus and the woman) usually outweigh the risks resulting from taking them during pregnancy.

Sexually Transmitted Diseases: Women who have a sexually transmitted disease may have problems during pregnancy. Chlamydial infection may cause preterm labor and premature rupture of the membranes containing the fetus. It can also cause conjunctivitis in newborns, as can gonorrhea. Syphilis in pregnant women may be transmitted to the fetus through the placenta. Syphilis can cause several birth defects.

✤ It's A Fact!!

Genital herpes can be transmitted to a baby during a vaginal delivery. A baby who is infected with herpes can develop a life-threatening brain infection called herpes encephalitis. If herpes produces sores in the genital area late in pregnancy, women are usually advised to give birth by cesarean section, so that the virus is not transmitted to the baby. If no sores are present, the risk of transmission is very low.

About one fourth of pregnant women who have untreated human immunodeficiency virus (HIV) infection, which causes AIDS, transmit it to their baby. Experts recommend that women with HIV infection take antiretroviral drugs during pregnancy. When pregnant women take these drugs, the risk of transmitting HIV to their baby is reduced to less than 2%. For some women with HIV infection, delivery by cesarean section, planned in advance, may further reduce the risk of transmitting HIV to the baby. Pregnancy does not seem to accelerate the progress of HIV infection in women.

Diabetes: For women who have diabetes before they become pregnant, the risks of complications during pregnancy depend on how long diabetes has been present and whether complications of diabetes, such as high blood pressure and kidney damage, are present. (In some women, diabetes develops during pregnancy; this disorder is called gestational diabetes.

The risk of complications during pregnancy can be reduced by controlling the level of sugar (glucose) in the blood. The level should be kept as nearly normal as possible throughout pregnancy. Measures to control the blood sugar level, such as diet, exercise, and insulin, should be started before pregnancy. Most pregnant women are asked to measure their blood sugar level several times a day at home. Controlling diabetes is particularly important late in pregnancy. Then, the blood sugar level tends to increase because the body becomes less responsive to insulin. A higher dose of insulin is usually needed.

When diabetes is poorly controlled later in pregnancy, the fetus is large, and the risk of stillbirth is increased. A large fetus is less likely to pass easily through the vagina and is more likely to be injured during vaginal delivery. Consequently, delivery by cesarean section is often necessary. The risk of preeclampsia (a type of high blood pressure that occurs during pregnancy) is also increased for women with diabetes.

The fetus's lungs tend to mature slowly. If an early delivery is being considered (for example, because the fetus is large), the doctor may remove and analyze a sample of the fluid that surrounds the fetus (amniotic fluid). This procedure, called amniocentesis, helps the doctor determine whether the fetus's lungs are mature enough for the newborn to breathe air.

For women with diabetes, the requirement for insulin drops dramatically immediately after delivery, but the requirement usually returns to what it was before pregnancy within about one week.

Liver And Gallbladder Disorders: Women who have chronic viral hepatitis or cirrhosis (scarring of the liver) are more likely to miscarry or to give birth prematurely. Cirrhosis can cause varicose veins to develop around the esophagus (esophageal varices). Pregnancy slightly increases the risk of massive bleeding from these veins, especially during the last three months of pregnancy.

Pregnant women who develop gallstones are closely monitored. If a gallstone blocks the gallbladder or causes an infection, surgery may be necessary. This surgery is usually safe for pregnant women and the fetus.

Asthma: In about half of the women who have asthma and become pregnant, the frequency or severity of asthma attacks does not change during pregnancy. About one fourth of the women improve during pregnancy, and about one fourth get worse. If pregnant women with severe asthma are treated with prednisone, the risk that the fetus will not grow as much as expected or will be born prematurely is increased.

Because asthma can change during pregnancy, doctors may ask women with asthma to use a peak flow meter to monitor their breathing more often. Pregnant women with asthma should see their doctor regularly so that treatment can be adjusted as needed. Maintaining good control of asthma is important. Inadequate treatment can result in serious problems. Cromolyn, bronchodilators (such as albuterol), and corticosteroids (such as beclomethasone) can be taken during pregnancy. Inhalation is the preferred way for taking these drugs. When inhaled, the drugs affect mainly the lungs and affect the whole body and the fetus less. Aminophylline (taken by mouth or given intravenously) and theophylline (taken by mouth) are occasionally used during pregnancy. Corticosteroids are taken by mouth only when other treatments are ineffective.

✔ **Quick Tip**

Being vaccinated against the influenza virus during the influenza (flu) season is particularly important for pregnant women with asthma.

Autoimmune Disorders: The abnormal antibodies produced in autoimmune disorders can cross the placenta and cause problems in the fetus. Pregnancy affects different autoimmune disorders in different ways.

Systemic Lupus Erythematosus (Lupus) may appear for the first time, worsen, or become less severe during pregnancy. How a pregnancy affects the course of lupus cannot be predicted, but the most common time for flare-ups is immediately after delivery.

Women who develop lupus often have a history of repeated miscarriages, fetuses that do not grow as much as expected, and preterm delivery. If women have complications due to lupus (such as kidney damage or high blood pressure), the risk of death for the fetus or newborn is increased.

In pregnant women, lupus antibodies may cross the placenta to the fetus. As a result, the fetus may have a very slow heart rate, anemia, a low platelet count, or a low white blood cell count. However, these antibodies gradually disappear over several weeks after the baby is born, and the problems they cause resolve except for the slow heart rate.

In **Graves' Disease**, antibodies stimulate the thyroid gland to produce excess thyroid hormone. These antibodies can cross the placenta and stimulate the thyroid gland in the fetus. As a result, the fetus may have a rapid heart rate and may not grow as much as expected. The fetus's thyroid gland may enlarge, forming a goiter. Very rarely, a goiter may be so large that it interferes with delivery through the vagina.

Usually, women with Graves' disease take the lowest possible effective dose of propylthiouracil, which slows the activity of the thyroid gland. Physical examinations and measurements of thyroid hormone levels are performed regularly because propylthiouracil crosses the placenta and may prevent the fetus from producing enough thyroid hormone. Often, Graves' disease becomes less severe during the third trimester, so the dose of propylthiouracil can be reduced or stopped. If necessary, the thyroid gland of pregnant women may be removed during the second trimester. These women must begin taking thyroid hormone 24 hours after surgery. Taking this hormone causes no problems for the fetus.

Myasthenia Gravis, which causes muscle weakness, does not usually cause serious or permanent complications during pregnancy. However, very rarely during labor, women who have myasthenia gravis may need help with breathing (assisted ventilation). The antibodies that cause this disorder can cross the placenta, so about one of five babies born to women with myasthenia gravis is born with the disorder. However, the resulting muscle weakness in the baby is usually temporary, because the antibodies from the mother gradually disappear and the baby does not produce antibodies of this type.

Idiopathic Thrombocytopenic Purpura can cause bleeding problems in pregnant women and their babies. If not treated during pregnancy, the disorder tends to become more severe. Corticosteroids, usually prednisone given by mouth, can increase the platelet count and improve blood clotting in pregnant women with this disorder. However, prednisone increases the risk that the fetus will not grow as much as expected or will be born prematurely.

High doses of gamma globulin may be given intravenously shortly before delivery. This treatment temporarily increases the platelet count and improves blood clotting. As a result, labor can proceed safely, and women can have a vaginal delivery without uncontrolled bleeding. Pregnant women are given platelet transfusions only when delivery by a cesarean section is needed or when the platelet count is so low that severe bleeding may occur. Rarely, when the platelet count remains dangerously low despite treatment, the spleen, which normally traps and destroys old blood cells and platelets, is removed. The best time for this surgery is during the second trimester.

The antibodies that cause the disorder may cross the placenta to the fetus, resulting rarely in a dangerously low platelet count before and immediately after birth. The baby may then bleed during labor and delivery and may, as a result, be injured or die, especially if bleeding occurs in the brain. The antibodies disappear within several weeks, and the baby's blood then clots normally.

Rheumatoid Arthritis does not affect the fetus, but delivery may be difficult for women if arthritis has damaged their hip joints or lower (lumbar) spine. The symptoms of rheumatoid arthritis may lessen during pregnancy, but they usually return to their original level after pregnancy.

Fibroids: Fibroids in the uterus, which are relatively common noncancerous tumors, may increase the risk of preterm labor, abnormal presentation of the fetus, a mislocated placenta (placenta previa), and repeated miscarriages. Rarely, fibroids interfere with the movement of the fetus through the vagina during labor.

Cancer: Because cancer tends to be life threatening and because delays in treatment may reduce the likelihood of successful treatment, cancer is usually treated the same way whether women are pregnant or not. Some of the usual treatments (surgery, chemotherapy drugs, and radiation therapy) may harm the fetus. Thus, some women may consider abortion. However, treatments can sometimes be timed so that risk to the fetus is reduced.

Chapter 27

Risk Factors That Develop During Pregnancy

During pregnancy, a problem may occur or a condition may develop to make the pregnancy high risk. For example, pregnant women may be exposed to something that can produce birth defects (teratogens), such as radiation, certain chemicals, drugs, or infections; or a disorder may develop. Some disorders are related to (are complications of) pregnancy.

Disorders That Develop During Pregnancy

During pregnancy, women may develop disorders that are not directly related to pregnancy. Some disorders increase the risk of problems for pregnant women or the fetus. They include disorders that cause a high fever, infections, and disorders that require abdominal surgery. Certain disorders are more likely to occur during pregnancy because of the many changes pregnancy causes in a woman's body. Examples are thromboembolic disease, anemia, and urinary tract infections.

Fevers: A disorder that causes a temperature greater than 103° F (39.5° C) during the first trimester increases the risk of a miscarriage and defects of

About This Chapter: Information in this chapter is excerpted from "Risk Factors That Develop During Pregnancy," *The Merck Manual of Medical Information—Second Home Edition*, pp. 1449–1456, edited by Mark H. Beers. Copyright 2003 by Merck & Co., Inc., Whitehouse Station, NJ. Reprinted with permission. The complete text of this material is available for free online at www.MerckManuals.com.

the brain or spinal cord in the baby. Fever late in pregnancy increases the risk of preterm labor.

Infections: Some infections that occur coincidentally during a pregnancy can cause birth defects. German measles (rubella) can cause birth defects, particularly of the heart and inner ear. Cytomegalovirus infection can cross the placenta and damage the fetus's liver and brain. Other viral infections that may harm the fetus or cause birth defects include herpes simplex and chickenpox (varicella). Toxoplasmosis, a protozoal infection, may cause miscarriage, death of the fetus, and serious birth defects. Listeriosis, a bacterial infection, can also harm the fetus. Bacterial infections of the vagina (such as bacterial vaginosis) during pregnancy may lead to preterm labor or premature rupture of the membranes containing the fetus. Treatment of infections with antibiotics may reduce the likelihood of these problems.

Disorders That Require Surgery: During pregnancy, a disorder that requires emergency surgery involving the abdomen may develop. This type of surgery increases the risk of preterm labor and can cause a miscarriage, especially early in pregnancy. Thus, surgery is usually delayed as long as possible unless the woman's long-term health may be affected.

If appendicitis develops during pregnancy, surgery to remove the appendix (appendectomy) is performed immediately because a ruptured appendix may be fatal. An appendectomy is not likely to harm the fetus or cause a miscarriage. However, appendicitis may be difficult to recognize during pregnancy. The cramping pain of appendicitis resembles uterine contractions, which are common during pregnancy. The appendix is pushed higher in the abdomen as the pregnancy progresses, so the location of pain due to appendicitis may not be what is expected.

If an ovarian cyst persists during pregnancy, surgery is usually postponed until after the 12th week of pregnancy. The cyst may be producing hormones that are supporting the pregnancy and often disappears without treatment. However, if a cyst or another mass is enlarging, surgery may be necessary before the 12th week. Such a mass may be cancerous.

Obstruction of the intestine during pregnancy can be very serious. If obstruction leads to gangrene of the intestine and peritonitis (inflammation of the membrane that lines the abdominal cavity), a woman may miscarry and her life is endangered. Exploratory surgery is usually performed promptly when pregnant women have symptoms of intestinal obstruction, particularly if they have had abdominal surgery or an abdominal infection.

Thromboembolic Disease: In the United States, thromboembolic disease is the leading cause of death in pregnant women. In thromboembolic disease, blood clots form in blood vessels. They may travel through the bloodstream and block an artery. The risk of developing thromboembolic disease is increased for about six to eight weeks after delivery. Most complications due to blood clots result from injuries that occur during delivery. The risk is much greater after a cesarean section than after vaginal delivery.

Blood clots usually form in the superficial veins of the legs as thrombophlebitis or in the deep veins as deep vein thrombosis. Symptoms include swelling, pain in the calves, and tenderness. The severity of the symptoms does not correlate with the severity of the disease. A clot can move from the legs to the lungs, where it may block one or more arteries in the lungs. This blockage, called pulmonary embolism, can be life threatening. If a clot blocks an artery supplying the brain, a stroke can result. Blood clots can also develop in the pelvis.

Women who have had a blood clot during a previous pregnancy may be given heparin (an anticoagulant) during subsequent pregnancies to prevent blood clots from forming. If women have symptoms suggesting a blood clot, Doppler ultrasonography may be performed to check for clots. If a blood clot is detected, heparin is started without delay. Heparin may be injected into a vein (intravenously) or under the skin (subcutaneously). Heparin does not cross the placenta and cannot harm the fetus. Treatment is continued for six to eight weeks after delivery, when the risk of blood clots is high. After delivery, warfarin may be used instead of heparin. Warfarin can be taken by mouth, has a lower risk of complications than heparin, and can be taken by women who are breastfeeding.

If pulmonary embolism is suspected, a lung ventilation and perfusion scan may be performed to confirm the diagnosis. This procedure involves injecting a tiny amount of a radioactive substance into a vein. The procedure is safe during pregnancy because the dose of the radioactive substance is so small. If the diagnosis of pulmonary embolism is still uncertain, pulmonary angiography is required.

Anemia: Most pregnant women develop some degree of anemia because they have an iron deficiency. The need for iron doubles during pregnancy, because iron is needed to make red blood cells in the fetus. Anemia may also develop during pregnancy because of a folic acid deficiency. Anemia can usually be prevented or treated by taking iron and folic acid supplements during pregnancy. However, if anemia becomes severe and persists, the blood's capacity to carry oxygen is decreased. As a result, the fetus may not receive enough oxygen, which is needed for normal growth and development, especially of the brain. Pregnant women who have severe anemia may become excessively tired, short of breath, and light-headed. The risk of preterm labor is increased. A normal amount of bleeding during labor and delivery can cause the anemia in these women to become dangerously severe. Women with anemia are more likely to develop infections after delivery. Also, if folic acid is deficient, the risk of having a baby with a birth defect of the brain or spinal cord, such as spina bifida, is increased.

Urinary Tract Infections: Urinary tract infections are common during pregnancy, probably because the enlarging uterus slows the flow of urine by pressing against the tubes that connect the kidneys to the bladder (ureters). When urine flow is slow, bacteria may not be flushed out of the urinary tract, increasing the risk of an infection. These infections increase the risk of preterm labor and premature rupture of the membranes containing the fetus. Sometimes an infection in the bladder or ureters spreads up the urinary tract and reaches a kidney, causing an infection there. Treatment consists of antibiotic therapy.

Pregnancy Complications

Pregnancy complications are problems that occur only during pregnancy. They may affect the woman, the fetus, or both and may occur at different times during the pregnancy. For example, complications such as a mislocated placenta (placenta previa) or premature detachment of the placenta from the uterus (placental abruption) can cause bleeding from the vagina during the last three months of pregnancy. Women who bleed at this time are at risk of losing the baby or of bleeding excessively (hemorrhaging) or dying during labor and delivery. However, most pregnancy complications can be effectively treated.

Some problems that result from hormonal changes during pregnancy cause only minor, transient symptoms in pregnant women. For example, the normal hormonal effects of pregnancy can slow the movement of bile through the bile ducts. Cholestasis of pregnancy may result. The most obvious symptom is itching all over the body (usually in the last few months of pregnancy). No rash develops. If itching is intense, cholestyramine may be given. The disorder usually resolves after delivery but tends to recur in subsequent pregnancies.

Hyperemesis Gravidarum: Hyperemesis gravidarum is extremely severe nausea and excessive vomiting during pregnancy. Hyperemesis gravidarum differs from ordinary morning sickness. If women vomit often and have nausea to such an extent that they lose weight and become dehydrated, they have hyperemesis gravidarum. If women vomit occasionally but gain weight and are not dehydrated, they do not have hyperemesis gravidarum. The cause of hyperemesis gravidarum is unknown.

Because hyperemesis gravidarum can be life threatening to pregnant women and the fetus, women who have it are hospitalized. An intravenous line is inserted into a vein to give fluids, sugar (glucose), electrolytes, and occasionally vitamins. Women who have this complication are not allowed to eat or drink anything for at least 24 hours. Sedatives, antiemetics, and other drugs are given as needed. After women are rehydrated and vomiting has subsided, they can begin eating frequent, small portions of bland foods. The size of the portions is increased if they can tolerate more food. Usually, vomiting stops within a few days. If symptoms recur, the treatment is repeated. Rarely, if weight loss continues and symptoms persist despite treatment, women are fed via a tube passed through the nose and down the throat to the small intestine for as long as necessary.

Preeclampsia: About 5% of pregnant women develop preeclampsia (toxemia of pregnancy). In this complication, an increase in blood pressure is accompanied by protein in the urine (proteinuria). Preeclampsia usually develops between the 20th week of pregnancy and the end of the first week after delivery. The cause of preeclampsia is unknown, but it is more common among women who are pregnant for the first time who are carrying two or more fetuses, who have had preeclampsia in a previous pregnancy, who already have high blood pressure or a blood vessel disorder, or who have sickle cell disease. It is also more common among girls aged 15 and younger and among women aged 35 and older.

A variation of severe preeclampsia, called the HELLP syndrome, occurs in some women. It consists of the following:

- hemolysis (the breakdown of red blood cells)

- elevated levels of liver enzymes, indicating liver damage

- low platelet count, making blood less able to clot, and increasing the risk of bleeding during and after labor

In 1 of 200 women who have preeclampsia, blood pressure becomes high enough to cause seizures; this condition is called eclampsia. One fourth of the cases of eclampsia occur after delivery, usually in the first two to four days. If not treated promptly, eclampsia may be fatal.

Preeclampsia may lead to premature detachment of the placenta from the uterus (placental abruption). Babies of women who have preeclampsia are four or five times more likely to have problems soon after birth than babies of women who do not have this complication. Babies may be small because the placenta malfunctions or because they are born prematurely.

If mild preeclampsia develops early in the pregnancy, bed rest at home may be sufficient, but such women should see their doctor frequently. If preeclampsia worsens, women are usually hospitalized. There, they are kept in bed and monitored closely until the fetus is mature enough to be delivered safely. Antihypertensives may be needed. A few hours before delivery, magnesium sulfate may be given intravenously to reduce the risk of seizures. If preeclampsia develops near the due date, labor is usually induced and the baby is delivered.

If preeclampsia is severe, the baby may be delivered by cesarean section, which is the quickest way, unless the cervix is already opened (dilated) enough for a prompt vaginal delivery. A prompt delivery reduces the risk of complications for women and the fetus. If blood pressure is high, drugs to lower blood pressure, such as hydralazine or labetalol, may be given intravenously before delivery is attempted. Treatment of the HELLP syndrome is usually the same as that of severe preeclampsia.

After delivery, women who have had preeclampsia or eclampsia are closely monitored for two to four days because they are at increased risk of seizures. As their condition gradually improves, they are encouraged to walk. They may remain in the hospital for a few days, depending on the severity of the preeclampsia and its complications. After returning home, these women may need to take drugs to lower blood pressure. Typically, they have a checkup at least every two weeks for the first few months after delivery. Their blood pressure may remain high for six to eight weeks. If it remains high longer, the cause may be unrelated to preeclampsia.

Rh Incompatibility: Rh incompatibility occurs when a pregnant woman has Rh-negative blood and the fetus has Rh-positive blood, inherited from a father who has Rh-positive blood. In about 13% of marriages in the United States, the man has Rh-positive blood and the woman has Rh-negative blood.

During a first pregnancy, Rh sensitization is unlikely, because no significant amount of the fetus's blood is likely to enter the woman's bloodstream until delivery; so the fetus or newborn rarely has problems. However, once a

♣ **It's A Fact!!**
Rh Sensitization

The Rh factor is a molecule that occurs on the surface of red blood cells of some people. Blood is Rh-positive if red blood cells have the Rh factor and Rh-negative if they do not. Problems can occur if the fetus's Rh-positive blood enters the woman's bloodstream. The woman's immune system may recognize the fetus's red blood cells as foreign and produce antibodies, called Rh antibodies, to destroy the fetus's red blood cells. The production of these antibodies is called Rh sensitization.

woman is sensitized, problems are more likely with each subsequent pregnancy in which the fetus's blood is Rh-positive. In each pregnancy, the woman produces Rh antibodies earlier and in larger amounts.

If Rh antibodies cross the placenta to the fetus, they may destroy some of the fetus's red blood cells. If red blood cells are destroyed faster than the fetus can produce new ones, the fetus can develop anemia. Such destruction is called hemolytic disease of the fetus (erythroblastosis fetalis) or of the newborn (erythroblastosis neonatorum). In severe cases, the fetus may die.

At the first visit to a doctor during a pregnancy, women are screened to determine whether they have Rh-positive or Rh-negative blood. If they have Rh-negative blood, their blood is checked for Rh antibodies, and the father's blood type is determined. If he has Rh-positive blood, Rh sensitization is a risk. In such cases, the blood of pregnant women is checked for Rh antibodies periodically during the pregnancy. The pregnancy can proceed as usual as long as no antibodies are detected.

If antibodies are detected, steps may be taken to protect the fetus, depending on how high the antibody level is. If the level becomes too high, amniocentesis may be performed. In this procedure, a needle is inserted through the skin to withdraw fluid from the amniotic sac. The level of bilirubin (a yellow pigment resulting from the normal breakdown of red blood cells) is measured in the fluid sample. If this level is too high, the fetus is given a blood transfusion. Usually, additional transfusions are given until the fetus is mature enough to be safely delivered; then labor is induced. The baby may need additional transfusions after birth. Sometimes no transfusions are needed until after birth.

As a precaution, women who have Rh-negative blood are given an injection of Rh antibodies at 28 weeks of pregnancy and within 72 hours after delivery of a baby who has Rh-positive blood, even after a miscarriage or an abortion. The antibodies given are called Rh0(D) immune globulin. This treatment destroys any red blood cells from the baby that may have entered the bloodstream of the women. Thus, there are no red blood cells from the baby to trigger the production of antibodies by these women, and subsequent pregnancies are usually not endangered.

Fatty Liver Of Pregnancy: This rare disorder occurs toward the end of pregnancy. The cause is unknown. Symptoms include nausea, vomiting, abdominal discomfort, and jaundice. The disorder may rapidly worsen, and liver failure may develop. Diagnosis is based on results of liver function tests and may be confirmed by a liver biopsy. The doctor may advise immediate termination of the pregnancy. The risk of death for pregnant women and the fetus is high, but those who survive recover completely. Usually, the disorder does not recur in subsequent pregnancies.

Peripartum Cardiomyopathy: The heart's walls may be damaged late in pregnancy or after delivery, causing peripartum cardiomyopathy. The cause is unknown. Peripartum cardiomyopathy tends to occur in women who have had several pregnancies, who are older, who are carrying twins, or who have preeclampsia. In some women, heart function does not return to normal after pregnancy. They may develop peripartum cardiomyopathy in subsequent pregnancies. These women should not become pregnant again. Peripartum cardiomyopathy can result in heart failure, which is treated.

Problems With Amniotic Fluid: Too much amniotic fluid (polyhydramnios) in the membranes containing the fetus (amniotic sac) stretches the uterus and puts pressure on the diaphragm of pregnant women. This complication can lead to severe breathing problems for the women or to preterm labor.

Too much fluid tends to accumulate when pregnant women have diabetes, are carrying more than one fetus (multiple pregnancy), or produce Rh antibodies to the fetus's blood. Another cause is birth defects in the fetus, especially a blocked esophagus or defects of the brain and spinal cord (such as spina bifida). About half the time, the cause is unknown.

Too little amniotic fluid (oligohydramnios) can also cause problems. If the amount of fluid is greatly reduced, the fetus's lungs may be immature, and the fetus may be compressed, resulting in deformities; this combination of conditions is called Potter syndrome.

Too little amniotic fluid tends to develop when the fetus has birth defects in the urinary tract, has not grown as much as expected, or dies. Other causes include the use of angiotensin-converting enzyme (ACE) inhibitors, such as enalapril or captopril, in the second and third trimesters. These drugs are given during pregnancy only when they must be used to treat severe heart failure or high blood pressure. Taking nonsteroidal anti-inflammatory drugs (NSAIDs) late in pregnancy can also reduce the amount of amniotic fluid.

Placenta Previa: Placenta previa is implantation of the placenta over or near the cervix, in the lower rather than the upper part of the uterus. The placenta may completely or partially cover the opening of the cervix. Placenta previa occurs in 1 of 200 deliveries, usually in women who have had more than one pregnancy or who have structural abnormalities of the uterus, such as fibroids.

Placenta previa can cause painless bleeding from the vagina that suddenly begins late in pregnancy. The blood may be bright red. Bleeding may become profuse, endangering the life of the woman and the fetus.

Ultrasonography helps doctors identify placenta previa and distinguish it from a placenta that has detached prematurely (placental abruption).

When bleeding is profuse, women may be hospitalized until delivery, especially if the placenta is located over the cervix. Women who bleed profusely may need repeated blood transfusions. When bleeding is slight and delivery is not imminent, doctors typically advise bed rest in the hospital. If the bleeding stops, women are usually encouraged to walk. If bleeding does not recur, they are usually sent home, provided that they can return to the hospital easily. A cesarean section is almost always performed before labor begins. If women with placenta previa go into labor, the placenta tends to become detached very early, depriving the baby of its oxygen supply. The lack of oxygen may result in brain damage or other problems in the baby.

Placental Abruption (Abruptio Placentae): Placental abruption is the premature detachment of a normally positioned placenta from the wall of the uterus. The placenta may detach incompletely (sometimes just 10 to 20%) or completely. The cause is unknown. Detachment of the placenta occurs in 0.4 to 3.5% of all deliveries. This complication is more common among women who have high blood pressure (including preeclampsia) and among women who use cocaine.

The uterus bleeds from the site where the placenta was attached. The blood may pass through the cervix and out the vagina as an external hemorrhage, or it may be trapped behind the placenta as a concealed hemorrhage. Symptoms depend on the degree of detachment and the amount of blood lost (which may be massive). Symptoms may include sudden continuous or crampy abdominal pain, tenderness when the abdomen is pressed, and shock. Premature detachment of the placenta can lead to widespread clotting inside the blood vessels (disseminated intravascular coagulation), kidney failure, and bleeding into the walls of the uterus, especially in pregnant women who also have preeclampsia. When the placenta detaches, the supply of oxygen and nutrients to the fetus may be reduced.

Doctors suspect premature detachment of the placenta on the basis of symptoms. Ultrasonography can confirm the diagnosis.

Women with premature detachment of the placenta are hospitalized. The usual treatment is bed rest. If symptoms lessen, women are encouraged to walk and may be discharged from the hospital. If bleeding continues or worsens (suggesting that the fetus is not getting enough oxygen), or if the pregnancy is near term, an early delivery is often best for the woman and the baby. If vaginal delivery is not possible, a cesarean section is performed.

Chapter 28

Ectopic Pregnancy

Ectopic means "out of place." In an ectopic pregnancy, a fertilized egg has implanted outside the uterus. The egg settles in the fallopian tubes more than 95% of the time. This is why ectopic pregnancies are commonly called "tubal pregnancies." The egg can also implant in the ovary, abdomen, or the cervix, so you may see these referred to as cervical or abdominal pregnancies.

None of these areas has as much space or nurturing tissue as a uterus for a pregnancy to develop. As the fetus grows, it will eventually burst the organ that contains it. This can cause severe bleeding and endanger the mother's life. A classical ectopic pregnancy never develops into a live birth.

What are the signs and symptoms?

Ectopic pregnancy can be difficult to diagnose because symptoms often mirror those of a normal early pregnancy. These can include missed periods, breast tenderness, nausea, vomiting, or frequent urination.

Pain is usually the first red flag. You might feel pain in your pelvis, abdomen, or, in extreme cases, even your shoulder or neck (if blood from a ruptured ectopic pregnancy builds up and irritates certain nerves). Most women

About This Chapter: This information was provided by KidsHealth, one of the largest resources online for medically reviewed health information written for parents, kids, and teens. For more articles like this one, visit www.KidsHealth.org, or www.TeensHealth.org. © 2004 The Nemours Foundation.

describe the pain as sharp and stabbing. It may concentrate on one side of the pelvis, and it may come and go or vary in intensity.

Any of the following additional symptoms can suggest an ectopic pregnancy:

- vaginal spotting or bleeding

- dizziness or fainting (caused by blood loss)

- low blood pressure (also caused by blood loss)

- lower back pain

What causes an ectopic pregnancy?

An ectopic pregnancy results from a fertilized egg's inability to work its way quickly enough down the fallopian tube into the uterus. An infection or inflammation of the tube may have partially or entirely blocked it. Pelvic inflammatory disease (PID) is the most common of these infections.

Endometriosis (when cells from the lining of the uterus detach and grow elsewhere in the body) or scar tissue from previous abdominal or fallopian surgeries can also cause blockages. More rarely, birth defects or abnormal growths can alter the shape of the tube and disrupt the egg's progress.

How is it diagnosed?

If you arrive in the emergency department complaining of abdominal pain, you'll likely be given a urine pregnancy test. Although these tests aren't sophisticated, they are fast—and speed can be crucial in treating ectopic pregnancy.

If you already know you're pregnant, or if the urine test comes back positive, you'll probably be given a quantitative hCG test. This blood test measures levels of the hormone human chorionic gonadotropin (hCG), which is produced by the placenta. The hormone hCG appears in the blood and urine as early as 10 days after conception, and its levels double every two days for the first ten weeks of pregnancy. If hCG levels are lower than expected for your stage of pregnancy, doctors are one step closer to diagnosing ectopic pregnancy.

The doctor will also give you a pelvic exam to locate the areas causing pain, to check for an enlarged, pregnant uterus, or to find any masses in your abdomen. You'll probably also get an ultrasound examination, which shows whether the uterus contains a developing fetus or if masses are present elsewhere in the abdominal area. But the ultrasound may not be able to detect every ectopic pregnancy.

A less commonly performed test, a culdocentesis, may be used to look for internal bleeding. In this test, a needle is inserted into the space at the very top of the vagina, behind the uterus and in front of the rectum. Any blood or fluid found there likely comes from a ruptured ectopic pregnancy.

Even with the best equipment, it's hard to see a pregnancy that's less than six weeks along. If your doctor can't diagnose ectopic pregnancy but can't rule it out, he or she may ask you to return every two days to measure your hCG levels. If these levels don't rise as quickly as they should, the doctor will continue to monitor you carefully until six weeks, when an ultrasound can be used.

What are the options for treatment?

Treatment of an ectopic pregnancy varies, depending on its size and location and whether you want the ability to conceive again.

An early ectopic pregnancy can sometimes be treated with an injection of methotrexate, which dissolves the fertilized egg and allows your body to reabsorb it. This nonsurgical approach minimizes scarring of your pelvic organs.

If the pregnancy is further along, you'll likely need surgery to remove the abnormal pregnancy. In the past, this was a major operation, requiring general anesthesia and a large incision across the pelvic area. This may still be necessary in cases of emergency or extensive internal injury.

However, the pregnancy may sometimes be removed using laparoscopy, a less invasive surgical procedure. The surgeon makes a small incision in the lower abdomen and then inserts a laparoscope. This long, hollow tube with a lighted end allows the doctor to view internal organs and insert other instruments as needed. Sometimes, a second small abdominal incision is made for the instruments. The ectopic pregnancy is then surgically removed and any damaged organs are repaired or removed. General or regional anesthesia may be used.

Whatever your treatment, the doctor will want to see you regularly afterward to make sure your hCG levels return to zero. This may take up to 12 weeks. An elevated hCG could mean that some ectopic tissue was missed. This tissue may have to be removed using methotrexate or additional surgery.

What about future pregnancies?

Approximately 30% of women who have had ectopic pregnancies will have difficulty becoming pregnant again. Your prognosis depends mainly on the extent of the damage and the surgery that was done.

If the fallopian tube has been spared, the chances of a future successful pregnancy is 60%. Even if one fallopian tube has been removed, the chances of having a successful pregnancy with the other tube can be greater than 40%.

The likelihood of a repeat ectopic pregnancy increases with each subsequent ectopic pregnancy.

Who's at risk for an ectopic pregnancy?

The risk of ectopic pregnancy is highest for women who are between 35 and 44 years old and have had the following:

- PID

- a previous ectopic pregnancy

- surgery on a fallopian tube

- infertility problems or medication to stimulate ovulation

> ♣ It's A Fact!!
> Once you have had one ectopic pregnancy, you face an approximate 15% chance of having another.

Some birth control methods can also increase your risk of ectopic pregnancy. If you get pregnant while using progesterone-only oral contraceptives, progesterone intrauterine devices (IUDs), or the morning-after pill, you're more likely to have an ectopic pregnancy.

When should you call your doctor?

If you believe you're at risk for an ectopic pregnancy, meet with your doctor to discuss your options before you become pregnant. There's nothing anyone can do to prevent ectopic pregnancy, but you can make sure it's detected early.

You and your doctor may want to plan on checking your hormone levels starting at ten days or scheduling an ultrasound at six weeks to ensure that your pregnancy is developing normally.

Call your doctor immediately if you're pregnant and experiencing any of the signs or symptoms of ectopic pregnancy. When it comes to detecting an ectopic pregnancy, "better safe than sorry" is more than just a cliché.

Chapter 29

Asthma During Pregnancy

Monitoring Asthma While You Are Pregnant

Early awareness of asthma symptoms and peak flow monitoring can help you and your doctor respond quickly to worsening of your asthma during pregnancy. It is important to identify and treat asthma symptoms before they become worse.

Asthma symptoms can range from mild to severe. It is important to identify and treat your asthma when the symptoms are still mild, so as to reduce the risk of a more serious episode. Common asthma symptoms may vary from person to person and include the following:

- cough
- shortness of breath
- tightness in the chest
- wheeze

Shortness of breath is common during pregnancy, and it may sometimes be difficult to tell if the cause is the increasing size of your baby or your asthma. A peak flow meter may enable you to tell the difference. A peak flow meter measures the airflow out of your lungs and can sometimes show a decrease hours, or even a day, before other asthma symptoms appear. Ask your doctor about using a peak flow meter to help monitor your asthma.

Asthma Action Plan For Your Pregnancy

When asthma symptoms and low peak flow numbers indicate your asthma is worsening, it is important to take action to ensure you and your baby receive enough oxygen. An asthma action plan is a written plan based on changes in asthma symptoms and peak flow numbers customized to your needs by your doctor to help you manage asthma worsening. It will give you information about when and how to use long-term control medicine and quick-relief medicine. It is a reminder of what to watch for and what steps to take so you will be able to make timely and appropriate decisions about managing your asthma during your pregnancy.

A small number of women with asthma may have an asthma episode severe enough to

☞ Remember!!
A severe asthma attack is a true medical emergency and you should seek medical assistance immediately.

be hospitalized so that you and your baby can be closely monitored. Your treatment may include oxygen, frequent inhaled medications, and intravenous (IV) steroids, all of which can be given without risk to your baby.

Asthma Management During Labor And Delivery

It is important to continue long-term control medicines and have quick-relief medicines available throughout labor and delivery. Bring your own medicine to the hospital so everyone will understand what you have been taking. The hospital will then provide whatever medication is needed.

Talk with your health care provider about pain control before your delivery date.

If anesthesia is required, spinal anesthesia is preferred to general ("gas") anesthesia. If you receive anesthesia of this form, you may be able to use your inhaled medicine as directed by your doctor.

If a cesarean section is required, you may need IV steroids.

Your breathing will be closely monitored as will your baby's heart rate with a fetal monitor to make sure that he or she is not showing signs of distress.

Plan ahead and discuss these decisions and potential problems with your health care providers. This will help decrease fears and problems that may arise once labor begins.

Breastfeeding When You Have Asthma

Research shows that breastfeeding for the first 6–12 months of life may help prevent or delay the development of certain allergies. The decision to breastfeed should be based on what you desire and your baby's needs.

In general when breastfeeding, the use of most asthma medicines does not affect your baby or interfere with your milk production. It is important to discuss your use of any medicines with your baby's doctor. Remember, your blood stream absorbs less medicine with inhaled medicine; therefore, less medicine passes into your breast milk.

The following list of medicines offers some additional information that can be discussed with your doctor:

- **Leukotriene Modifiers:** The leukotriene modifiers are excreted in breast milk. Because the safety of these drugs has not been confirmed, they should not be taken while you are breastfeeding.

- **Oral Steroids:** Oral steroids pass through breast milk in trace amounts. Even at high dosages, these drugs have not been associated with problems.

- **Theophylline:** This medicine passes through breast milk in trace amounts. This has been associated with irritability and insomnia in some infants.

By all means, do not resume cigarette smoking after your baby is born. The toxic substances of cigarettes can be transmitted through breastfeeding as well as by the inhalation of second hand smoke.

Remember that good asthma management is important for you and your baby. Talk with your doctor and other healthcare providers about any questions or concerns you have.

Chapter 30

Diabetes And Pregnancy

Diabetes: An Overview

Diabetes is often detected in women during their childbearing years and can affect the health of both the mother and her unborn child. Poor control of diabetes in a woman who is pregnant increases the chances for birth defects and other problems for the baby. It might cause serious complications for the woman also.

Will my baby have diabetes?

Babies born to mothers with diabetes do not come into the world with diabetes. However, if the mother's diabetes was not controlled during pregnancy, the baby can very quickly develop low blood sugar after birth and must be watched very closely until his or her body adjusts the amount of insulin it makes.

What can happen to a woman with type 1 or type 2 diabetes that becomes pregnant?

Out of control blood sugar could lead to a woman having a miscarriage. Out of control blood sugar might also cause high blood pressure in

About This Chapter: Information under the heading "Diabetes: An Overview" is excerpted from "Diabetes and Pregnancy Frequently Asked Questions," Centers for Disease Control and Prevention (CDC), October 2005. Text under the heading "Gestational Diabetes" is from "What I Need To Know About Gestational Diabetes," National Diabetes Information Clearinghouse (NDIC), a service of the National Institute of Diabetes and Digestive and Kidney Diseases (NIDDK), NIH Publication No. 06-5129, April 2006.

a woman during pregnancy. High blood pressure during pregnancy might lead to a baby being born early and also could cause seizures or a stroke in the woman during labor and delivery. Sometimes, out of control blood sugar causes a woman to make extra large amounts of amniotic fluid around the baby, which might lead to preterm (early) labor. Another problem common to a pregnant woman with uncontrolled diabetes is that her baby grows too large. Besides causing discomfort to the woman during the last few months of pregnancy, an extra large baby can lead to problems during delivery for both the mother and the baby.

> ♣ **It's A Fact!!**
>
> Diabetes in the father does not affect the developing baby during pregnancy. However, depending on the type of diabetes the father has, the baby might have a greater chance of developing diabetes later in life.
>
> Source: Centers for Disease Control and Prevention (CDC)

What can happen to the baby of a woman with type 1 or type 2 diabetes during pregnancy?

A woman who has diabetes that is not tightly controlled has a higher chance of having a baby with a birth defect. The organs of the baby form during the first two months of pregnancy, often before a woman knows that she is pregnant. Out of control blood sugar can affect those organs while they are being formed and cause serious birth defects or can lead to miscarriage of the developing baby.

If the woman's blood sugar remains out of control throughout the pregnancy, the baby likely will grow extra large. The extra large baby can cause problems during and after delivery.

If the woman with diabetes has problems that lead to a preterm birth, the baby might have breathing problems, heart problems, bleeding into the brain, intestinal problems, and vision problems. A woman with diabetes might have a baby born on time with low birth weight. A baby with low birth weight might have problems with eating, gaining weight, fighting off infections, and staying warm.

Gestational Diabetes

What is gestational diabetes?

Gestational (jes-TAY-shun-ul) diabetes is diabetes that is found for the first time when a woman is pregnant. Diabetes means that your blood glucose (also called blood sugar) is too high. Your body uses glucose for energy, but too much glucose in your blood can be harmful. When you are pregnant, too much glucose is not good for your baby.

What causes gestational diabetes?

Changing hormones and weight gain are part of a healthy pregnancy, but both changes make it hard for your body to keep up with its need for a hormone called insulin. When that happens, your body doesn't get the energy it needs from the food you eat.

What is my risk of gestational diabetes?

If you have any of the following risk factors, ask your health care team about testing for gestational diabetes.

- I have a parent, brother, or sister with diabetes.

- I am African American, American Indian, Asian American, Hispanic/ Latino, or Pacific Islander.

- I am 25 years old or older.

- I am overweight.

- I have had gestational diabetes before, or I have given birth to at least one baby weighing more than 9 pounds.

- I have been told that I have "pre-diabetes," a condition in which blood glucose levels are higher than normal, but not yet high enough for a diagnosis of diabetes. Other names for it are "impaired glucose tolerance" and "impaired fasting glucose."

How is gestational diabetes diagnosed?

Your health care team will check your blood glucose level. Depending on your risk and your test results, you may have one or more of the following tests.

Fasting Blood Glucose Or Random Blood Glucose Test: Your doctor may check your blood glucose level using a test called a fasting blood glucose test. Before this test, your doctor will ask you to fast, which means having nothing to eat or drink except water for at least 8 hours; or your doctor may check your blood glucose at any time during the day. This is called a random blood glucose test.

> ✤ **It's A Fact!!**
>
> Out of every 100 pregnant women in the United States, three to eight get gestational diabetes.
>
> Source: National Diabetes Information Clearinghouse (NDIC)

Screening Glucose Challenge Test: For this test, you will drink a sugary beverage and have your blood glucose level checked an hour later. This test can be done at any time of the day.

Oral Glucose Tolerance Test: If you have this test, your health care provider will give you special instructions to follow. For at least 3 days before the test, you should eat normally. Then you will fast for at least 8 hours before the test.

The health care team will check your blood glucose level before the test. Then you will drink a sugary beverage. The staff will check your blood glucose levels 1 hour, 2 hours, and 3 hours later. If your levels are above normal at least twice during the test, you have gestational diabetes.

How will gestational diabetes affect my baby?

Untreated or uncontrolled gestational diabetes can mean problems for your baby. Your baby might be born very large and with extra fat; this can make delivery difficult and more dangerous for your baby. Your baby might also have low blood glucose right after birth or have breathing problems.

If you have gestational diabetes, your health care team may recommend an ultrasound exam to see how your baby is growing, use "kick counts" to check your baby's activity (the time between the baby's movements), or do special "stress" tests.

Both you and your baby are at increased risk for type 2 diabetes for the rest of your lives.

How will gestational diabetes affect me?

Gestational diabetes may do the following:

- increase your risk of high blood pressure during pregnancy

- increase your risk of a large baby and the need for cesarean section at delivery

The good news is your gestational diabetes will probably go away after your baby is born. You may also get gestational diabetes again if you get pregnant again.

How is gestational diabetes treated?

Treating gestational diabetes means taking steps to keep your blood glucose levels in a target range. You will learn how to control your blood glucose by using a meal plan, having regular physical activity, and using insulin if needed.

Meal Plan: You will talk with a dietitian or a diabetes educator who will design a meal plan to help you choose foods that are healthy for you and your baby.

You may be advised to do the following:

- Limit sweets.

- Eat three small meals and one to three snacks every day.

- Be careful about when and how much carbohydrate-rich food you eat. Your meal plan will tell you when to eat carbohydrates and how much to eat at each meal and snack.

- Include fiber in your meals in the form of fruits, vegetables, and whole-grain crackers, cereals, and bread.

Physical Activity: Physical activity, such as walking and swimming, can help you reach your blood glucose targets. Talk with your health care team about the type of activity that is best for you. If you are already active, tell your health care team what you do.

Insulin: Some women with gestational diabetes need insulin, in addition to a meal plan and physical activity, to reach their blood glucose targets. If necessary, your health care team will show you how to give yourself insulin. Insulin is not harmful for your baby. It cannot move from your bloodstream to the baby's.

How will I know whether my blood glucose levels are on target?

Your health care team may ask you to use a small device called a blood glucose meter to check your levels on your own. You will learn how to use the meter, how to prick your finger to obtain a drop of blood, what your target range is, and when to check your blood glucose. You may be asked to check your blood glucose when you wake up, just before meals, 1 or 2 hours after breakfast, 1 or 2 hours after lunch, and 1 or 2 hours after dinner.

Each time you check your blood glucose, write down the results in a record book. Take the book with you when you visit your health care team. If your results are often out of range, your health care team will suggest ways you can reach your targets.

Will I need to do other tests on my own?

Your health care team may teach you how to test for ketones (KEE-tones) in your morning urine or in your blood. High levels of ketones are a sign that your body is using your body fat for energy instead of the food you eat. Using fat for energy is not recommended during pregnancy. Ketones may be harmful for your baby.

If your ketone levels are high, your health care providers may suggest that you change the type or amount of food you eat; or you may need to change your meal times or snack times.

After I have my baby, how can I find out whether my diabetes is gone?

You will probably have a blood glucose test 6 to 12 weeks after your baby is born to see whether you still have diabetes. For most women, gestational diabetes goes away after pregnancy. You are, however, at risk of having gestational diabetes during future pregnancies or getting type 2 diabetes later.

> ✔ **Quick Tip**
>
> Remind your health care team to check your blood glucose levels regularly. Women who have had gestational diabetes should continue to be tested for diabetes or pre-diabetes every 1 to 2 years. Diagnosing diabetes or pre-diabetes early can help prevent complications such as heart disease later.
>
> Source: National Diabetes Information Clearinghouse (NDIC)

Chapter 31

Eating Disorders And Pregnancy

Pregnancy and motherhood. Professionals recommend that women with eating disorders do their best to resolve the eating disorder related weight and behavior problems before they attempt to get pregnant.

Pregnancy and motherhood require a great amount of physical and psychological strength. During pregnancy, the growing baby receives all its nourishment from the mother's body. When stores of carbohydrates, proteins, fats, vitamins, minerals, and other nutrients are low, a woman's body will drain them to support the growth and development of the baby. If reserves are not sufficiently restored through healthy eating, the mother can become severely malnourished, and this in turn can lead to depression, exhaustion, and many other serious health complications.

The average woman gains between 25–35 pounds during pregnancy. While this amount is required for a healthy pregnancy, for women with eating disorders, having to gain this amount can be very frightening. Some women with disordered eating are able to more easily cope with weight gain during pregnancy because they see it as a sacrifice for an important cause. But others may plunge into deep depression as they struggle with the tension between the idea of weight gain and their body image issues. Most women with eating disorders fall somewhere between these two extremes.

About This Chapter: Information in this chapter is from "Eating Disorders and Pregnancy: Some Facts about the Risks," © 2005 National Eating Disorders Association. Reprinted with permission. For additional information, visit www.NationalEatingDisorders.org, or call the toll-free Information and Referral Helpline at 800-931-2237.

♣ It's A Fact!!
Pregnancy And Pica: Non-Food Cravings

Pica is the practice of craving substances with little or no nutritional value. Most pica cravings involve non-food substances such as dirt or chalk. The word pica is Latin for magpie, which is a bird notorious for eating almost anything.

It is true that the majority of women will experience cravings during pregnancy; however, most of these cravings are for things like pickles and ice cream. Pica cravings are most commonly seen in children and occur in approximately 25–30% of all children; pica cravings in pregnant women are even less common.

What causes pica during pregnancy? The reason that some women develop pica cravings during pregnancy is not known for certain. There is currently no identified cause; however, according to the *Journal of American Dietetic Association*, there may be a connection to an iron deficiency.

Some speculate that pica cravings are the body's attempt to obtain vitamins or minerals that are missing through normal food consumption. Sometimes pica cravings may be related to an underlying physical or mental illness.

What are typical pica cravings during pregnancy? The most common substances craved during pregnancy are dirt, clay, and laundry starch. Other pica cravings include burnt matches, stones, charcoal, mothballs, ice, cornstarch, toothpaste, soap, sand, plaster, coffee grounds, baking soda, and cigarette ashes.

Are pica cravings harmful to the baby? Eating non-food substances is potentially harmful to both you and your baby. Eating non-food substances may interfere with the nutrient absorption of healthy food substances and actually cause a deficiency. Pica cravings are also a concern because non-food items may contain toxic or parasitic ingredients.

What can you do if you have pica cravings? Don't panic; it happens and is not abnormal. The most important thing is to inform your health care provider to make sure you have a complete understanding of the specific risks associated with your cravings. Here are some suggestions to help you deal with pica cravings:

• Inform your health care provider and review your prenatal health records.

• Monitor your iron status along with other vitamin and mineral intake.

• Consider potential substitutes for the cravings such as chewing sugarless gum.

• Inform a friend of your craving who can help you avoid non-food items.

Source: Reprinted with permission from the American Pregnancy Association, http://www.americanpregnancy.org, © 2006. All rights reserved.

The Relationship Between Specific Eating Disorders And Pregnancy

Women with anorexia nervosa are underweight and may not gain enough weight during pregnancy. They risk having a baby with abnormally low birth weight and related health problems. Women with bulimia nervosa, who continue to purge, may suffer dehydration, chemical imbalances, or even cardiac irregularities. Pregnancy heightens these health risks. Women who are overweight due to binge eating are at greater risk of developing high blood pressure, gestational diabetes, and overgrown babies.

Risks For The Mother: Poor nutrition, dehydration, cardiac irregularities, gestational diabetes, severe depression during pregnancy, premature births, labor complications, difficulties nursing, and post-partum depression.

Risks For The Baby: Poor development, premature birth, low birth weight for age, respiratory distress, other perinatal complications, and feeding difficulties.

Professionals recommend that women with eating disorders do their best to resolve the eating disorder related weight and behavior problems before they attempt to get pregnant. It is important to consult with your physician, counselors, and/or registered dietitian before attempting to get pregnant. Women with eating disorders who become pregnant are advised to seek specialized medical and psychological help. Pregnant women with eating disorders should inform their obstetricians about these problems and may require "high risk" obstetrical care.

Remember, eat healthy, well-balanced meals and maintain a healthy weight for several months before conceiving and throughout pregnancy to protect the health of yourself and your baby.

What If I Become Pregnant While Struggling With An Eating Disorder?

Though having an eating disorder may decrease the chances of pregnancy, sometimes women with anorexia or bulimia do become pregnant. When this happens, steps should be taken to protect the health of the mother and the baby. Professionals can address the specific needs related to pregnancy and disordered eating only if you are willing to be completely honest with them about your struggles.

If you are pregnant and struggling with disordered eating, the following will apply to you:

- Be honest with your prenatal health provider regarding past or present struggles with an eating disorder or disordered eating.

- Extra appointments with your prenatal health provider may be necessary to more closely track the growth and development of your baby.

- Consult a nutritionist with expertise in eating disorders before or immediately after becoming pregnant. Work with the nutritionist throughout the pregnancy to create a plan for healthy eating and weight gain. Continue to see her post-partum. She can help you return to a normal weight through healthy means.

- Individual counseling during and after pregnancy can help you cope with your concerns and fears regarding food, weight gain, body image, and the new role of mothering.

- Attend a support group for people with eating disorders.

- If your doctor approves, attend a prenatal exercise class. It can help you practice healthy limits to exercising.

- Other classes on pregnancy, childbirth, child development, and parenting skills can also be helpful in preparing to become a mother.

- Allow your prenatal health provider to weigh you. This information is essential to track the health of your baby. If you would prefer not to monitor your weight gain, ask your doctor about standing on the scale backwards.

- Under certain circumstances, for example if you suffer from severe depression or obsessive-compulsive problems, you may require medications for these conditions even during pregnancy.

The skills and support of a multidisciplinary team of health care providers and of family and friends can help you deliver a healthy baby and protect yourself.

Chapter 32

Multiple Births

A multiple gestation is a pregnancy in which a woman is carrying two or more babies (fetuses). In the past two decades, the number of multiple births in the United States has jumped dramatically. Between 1980 and 2000, the number of twin births has increased 74 percent, and the number of higher order multiples (triplets or more) has increased fivefold, according to the National Center for Health Statistics.

The rising number of multiple gestations is a concern because women who are expecting more than one baby are at increased risk of certain pregnancy complications including preterm delivery (before 37 completed weeks of pregnancy). Babies who are born preterm are at risk of serious health problems during the newborn period as well as lasting disabilities and death.

Some of the complications associated with multiple gestations can be minimized or prevented when they are diagnosed early. There are a number of steps a pregnant woman and her health care provider can take to help improve the chances that her babies will be born healthy.

Why are multiple gestations increasing?

About one-third of the increase in multiple gestations is due to the fact that more women over age 30 (who are more likely to conceive multiples) are having babies. The remainder of the increase is due to the use of fertility-stimulating drugs and assisted reproductive techniques (ART) such as in vitro fertilization (IVF) (in which eggs are removed from the mother, fertilized in a laboratory dish, and then transferred to the uterus). According to the most recent survey of ART programs in the United States, 56 percent of births resulting from these procedures were multiples.

♣ **It's A Fact!!**
Today, about 3 percent of babies in this country are born in sets of two, three or more, and about 95 percent of these multiple births are twins.

Doctors now realize that it is crucial to monitor fertility treatments so that women will have fewer, but healthier, babies. This involves limiting the number of embryos transferred during IVF or halting treatment with fertility drugs during a cycle if ultrasound shows that a large number of eggs could be released. In fact, the rate of higher-order multiple births has declined slightly in the past two years.

How are multiple gestations diagnosed?

Although previous generations often were surprised by the delivery of twins (or other multiples), today most parents-to-be learn the news fairly early. An ultrasound examination can detect more than 95 percent of multiples by the beginning of the second trimester. (Sometimes a seemingly normal twin gestation that is identified very early is later found to have only one fetus. These so-called "vanishing twin" events are not well understood.)

An abnormal result on the triple or quadruple screen—blood tests done around the 16th week of pregnancy to identify babies at increased risk of certain birth defects—also alerts a health care provider to the possibility of multiples, as does hearing more than one fetal heartbeat during a routine examination. A provider also may suspect that a woman is carrying more than one baby if she puts on weight more rapidly than anticipated in the first trimester, her uterus is larger than expected, or if she has severe pregnancy-related nausea and vomiting (morning sickness). Some women also may notice more fetal movement than in a previous singleton pregnancy. Whenever a multiple gestation is suspected, the health care provider will most likely recommend an ultrasound examination to find out for sure.

What complications occur more frequently in a multiple gestation?

Twins generally face the fewest medical complications and are usually born healthy. The more babies a woman carries at once, the greater her risk of complications.

Close to 60 percent of twins, over 90 percent of triplets, and virtually all quadruplets and higher multiples are born preterm. The length of gestation decreases with each additional baby. On average, most singleton pregnancies last 39 weeks; for twins, 36 weeks; for triplets, 32 weeks; for quadruplets, 30 weeks; and for quintuplets, 29 weeks.

Most preterm multiples weigh less than 5 1/2 pounds (2,500 grams), which is considered low birth weight. Low birth weight babies, especially those born before 32 weeks of gestation and/or weighing less than 3 1/3 pounds (1,500 grams), are at increased risk of health complications in the newborn period as well as lasting disabilities such as mental retardation, cerebral palsy, and vision and hearing loss. While advances in caring for very small infants has brightened the outlook for these tiny babies, chances remain slim that all infants in a set of sextuplets or more will survive and thrive.

Before birth, identical twins face an additional risk. One-third of all twin pairs are identical—they begin as one fertilized egg that subsequently divides in half. The remaining two-thirds of twins are fraternal, resulting from two different eggs fertilized by two different sperm. Fraternal twins are no more similar genetically than are any other siblings. They may not be the same sex; they may not even look alike. Higher order multiples can result from three (or more) eggs being fertilized, one egg splitting twice (or more), or a combination of both.

Identical twin fetuses have a 15 percent chance of developing a serious complication called twin-to-twin transfusion syndrome. This condition, which occurs when there is a connection between the two babies' blood

---

♣ It's A Fact!!

A woman also has a higher-than-average chance of conceiving twins if she has a personal or family history of fraternal (non-identical) twins or if she is obese.

vessels in their shared placenta, can result in one baby getting too much blood flow and the other too little. Until recently, severe cases often resulted in the loss of both babies. Recent studies, though, suggest that the use of amniocentesis to drain off excess fluid can save about 60 percent of affected babies. Removing the excess fluid appears to improve blood flow in the placenta and reduces the risk of preterm labor. Recent studies also suggest that using laser surgery to seal off the connection between the blood vessels may save a similar number of babies. An advantage of laser surgery is that only one treatment is needed, while amniocentesis generally must be repeated more than once.

Women who are pregnant with multiples also face an increased risk of pregnancy-related forms of high blood pressure (preeclampsia) and diabetes. More than half of triplet pregnancies are complicated by preeclampsia. With proper treatment, these disorders usually do not pose a major risk to mother or baby.

Should a woman expecting multiples gain extra weight?

Eating right and gaining the recommended amount of weight reduces the risk of having a low birth weight baby in singleton, as well as multiple, gestations. A healthy weight gain is especially important if a woman is pregnant with twins or more, as multiples have a higher risk of preterm birth and low birth weight than singletons.

Women who begin pregnancy at a normal weight and who are expecting one baby usually are advised to gain 25 to 35 pounds over nine months. Women of normal weight who are expecting twins are usually advised to gain 35 to 45 pounds. Women pregnant with triplets should probably aim for a gain of 50 to 60 pounds.

Studies show that gaining enough weight in the first 20 to 24 weeks of pregnancy is especially important for women carrying multiples. In a twin pregnancy, a gain of at least 24 pounds by the 24th week of pregnancy helps reduce the risk of having preterm and low birth weight babies. A good early weight gain may be especially important in multiple gestations because these pregnancies tend to be shorter than singleton pregnancies. Studies also suggest that a good early weight gain aids in development of the placenta, possibly improving its ability to pass along nutrients to the babies.

The American College of Obstetricians and Gynecologists recommends that women with multiple pregnancies consume about 300 more calories a day than women carrying one baby (a total of about 2,700 to 2,800 calories a day). However, women pregnant with multiples should discuss the number of extra calories they should eat with their health care providers. They also should take a prenatal vitamin that is recommended by their health care provider and that contains at least 30 milligrams of iron. Iron deficiency anemia is common in multiple gestations, and it can increase the risk of preterm delivery.

What special care is needed in a multiple gestation?

Women who are expecting multiples generally need to visit their health care providers more frequently than women expecting one baby to help prevent, detect, and treat the complications that develop more often in a multiple gestation. Health care providers usually recommend twice-monthly visits during the second trimester and weekly (or more frequent) visits during the third trimester.

Starting around the 20th week of pregnancy, a health care provider will monitor the pregnant woman carefully for signs of preterm labor. She may do an internal exam or recommend a vaginal ultrasound examination to see if the woman's cervix is shortening (a possible sign that labor may begin soon). Some providers also do electronic uterine monitoring. Home uterine monitoring was once recommended for women at especially high risk of preterm labor, but studies of women expecting twins did not find it useful.

When a woman develops preterm labor, her provider may recommend bed rest in the hospital and, possibly, treatment with drugs that may postpone labor. If the provider does not believe labor will stop, and if the babies are likely to be born before 34 weeks gestation, she will probably recommend that the pregnant woman be treated with drugs called corticosteroids. These drugs help speed fetal lung development and reduce the likelihood and severity of breathing and other problems during the newborn period.

Even if a woman pregnant with twins has no signs of preterm labor, her provider may recommend cutting back on activities sometime between the 20th and 30th weeks of pregnancy. She may be advised to cut back on activities even sooner and to rest several times a day if she is expecting more than two babies.

As a multiple gestation progresses, the health care provider will regularly check the pregnant woman's blood pressure for preeclampsia. Regular ultrasound examinations often are recommended to check on the babies' rates of growth including growth differences among them, which can be signs of serious problems. During the third trimester, the provider may recommend tests of fetal well-being (such as the non-stress test, which measures fetal heart rate when the baby is moving).

Can a woman expecting multiples deliver vaginally?

While the chance of a cesarean delivery is higher in twin than in singleton births, about half of women expecting twins can have a normal vaginal delivery. Chances are good if both babies are in a normal, head-down position. However, when a woman is carrying three or more babies, a cesarean delivery is usually recommended because it is safer for the babies.

Chapter 33

Preterm Birth

What Is Preterm Labor?

In most pregnancies, labor starts between 38 and 42 weeks after the last menstrual period. Labor is considered preterm labor when it starts before the beginning of the 37th week.

Labor starts with regular contractions of the uterus. The cervix thins out (effaces) and opens up (dilates) so the baby can enter the birth canal. It is not known exactly what causes labor to start. Hormones produced by both the woman and fetus play a role. Changes in the uterus, which may be caused by these hormones, may cause labor to start.

Why The Concern?

Preterm birth accounts for about 75% of newborn deaths that are not related to birth defects. Growth and development in the last part of pregnancy is critical to the baby's health. The earlier the baby is born, the greater the risk of problems.

Preterm babies (also called premature babies or "preemies") tend to grow more slowly. They may have problems with their eyes, ears, breathing, and

About This Chapter: Information in this chapter is from "Preterm Labor." Reprinted with permission from the University of Michigan Health System, www.med.umich.edu. Copyright © 2005 Regents of the University of Michigan.

nervous system. School, learning, and behavior problems are more common in children who were preterm babies.

Signs Of Preterm Labor

If preterm labor is found early enough, delivery can sometimes be prevented or postponed. This will give your baby extra time to grow and mature. Even a few more days may mean a healthier baby.

Sometimes the signs that preterm labor may be starting are fairly easy to detect. The warning signs of preterm labor are listed below. If you have any of these signs, do not wait. Call your health care provider.

♣ **It's A Fact!!**

Preterm labor may be a normal process that starts early for some reason; or, it may be started by some other problem, like infection of the uterus or amniotic fluid. In most cases of preterm labor, the exact cause is not known.

- watery vaginal discharge (enough to make your underwear wet)

- any vaginal bleeding before 37 weeks

- if you experience any of the following for four to six hours or longer: pelvic or lower abdominal pressure; constant, low, dull backache; mild abdominal cramps like a menstrual period, with or without diarrhea; regular contractions or uterine tightening, often painless

- ruptured membranes (your "water breaks")

Constant backache or pressure without any other signs is not likely to be preterm labor.

If you are having contractions, do the following:

- Drink 16 oz. of a non-caffeinated beverage, lie down, turn onto your side, and count the contractions for an hour.

- If your contractions are occurring more than once every ten minutes (six or more per hour), call your health care provider or nurse right away.

- If you have had very short labors before, call sooner—do not wait.

Diagnosing Preterm Labor

It can be hard to tell the difference between true and false labor. Preterm labor can only be diagnosed by finding changes in the cervix. It is common for women to have contractions before labor starts, sometimes called Braxton Hicks contractions or false labor. These may be painful and regular but usually go away within an hour or with rest. If you have contractions more often than six times an hour that continue for more than an hour, call your health care provider right away.

Fetal monitoring is used to record the heartbeat of the fetus and contractions of your uterus. You may be watched for a time and then examined again to see whether your cervix changes.

Women At Risk

Some women are at greater risk for preterm labor than others. Women who have little or no prenatal care and those who have had preterm labor before are at increased risk. Preterm labor can happen to anyone, however, without warning.

A number of other factors have also been linked to preterm labor. There are also factors linked to the fetus that make preterm labor more likely. For instance, too much fluid in the amniotic sac that surrounds the baby is a risk factor. Problems with the placenta or certain birth defects also increase the risk. You may be at risk for preterm labor if any of the following factors apply to you:

- You have warning signs of preterm labor.
- You have had preterm labor during this pregnancy.
- You had preterm labor or preterm birth in a previous pregnancy.
- You are carrying more than one baby (twins, triplets).
- You have had one or more second-trimester induced abortions (the planned ending of a pregnancy).
- You have an abnormal cervix (due to surgery, for example).
- You have an abnormal uterus.
- You have had abdominal surgery during this pregnancy.

- You have had a serious infection while pregnant.

- You have had bleeding in the second or third trimester of your pregnancy.

- You are underweight or you weigh less than 100 pounds.

- You smoke or use cocaine.

- You have had little or no prenatal care.

Despite what is known about these risk factors, much remains to be learned about preterm labor. Half of the women who go into preterm labor have no known risk factors.

If you are at risk for preterm labor, you may be advised to take certain steps to lower the risk of preterm birth. These steps may involve changing your life style, having more frequent visits with your health care provider, and learning how to monitor your contractions.

If you are at risk for preterm labor, be sure to get early prenatal care, eat well, and get enough rest. You may need to see your health care provider more often for exams and tests. You should give up unhealthy habits, such as drinking alcohol and smoking cigarettes. Stay away from drugs other than those prescribed by your health care provider.

Women at risk for preterm labor usually do not have to give up their jobs unless preterm labor has actually been diagnosed. You may be advised to avoid prolonged standing, heavy lifting, or other hard or tiring tasks during pregnancy. If you take childbirth preparation classes, you should tell the teacher you are at risk for preterm labor. He or she may advise you to skip certain exercises. Women at risk may also be advised to cut down on travel. Ask your health care provider about any other changes you may need to make in your daily routine.

If you have a history of preterm labor or birth, or have signs of preterm labor, you may wonder about having sex during pregnancy. Many women worry that the uterine contractions that often follow sex and orgasm will lead to preterm labor. Although in most cases the contractions stop, these are natural and realistic concerns that should be discussed with both your partner and your health care provider. You may be advised to restrict sexual activity or to monitor yourself for contractions after sex. Your health care provider may also ask that your partner use a condom during sex to lower the risk of infection.

Stopping Labor

Your health care provider may try to stop preterm labor a number of ways.

Monitoring For Contractions

After about 20 weeks of pregnancy, you may be asked to monitor yourself for signs of uterine activity or tightening. To monitor yourself, lie down and gently feel the entire surface of your lower abdomen with your fingertips. This is called palpation. You are feeling for a firm tightening over the surface of your uterus. Usually these feelings of tightening are not painful.

> **☞ Remember!!**
>
> A diagnosis of preterm labor can be made only after a pelvic exam to see whether your cervix has begun to change. You should contact your health care provider each time you have more than six contractions per hour, unless he or she has advised otherwise.

If you feel contractions, turn onto your side and keep monitoring for an hour. Keep track of when each contraction starts and ends and the total number in one hour. If you have had very short labors before, you should call your health care provider sooner—do not wait. Having some uterine activity before 37 weeks of pregnancy is normal; but if your contractions are occurring more than once every ten minutes (six or more per hour), you need to call your health care provider right away. You may be in preterm labor.

Treatment

Sometimes labor can be stopped. Other times, the baby must be delivered. Your health care provider may try to stop labor if the following is true:

- It is detected early enough.

- You or your baby are not in danger from infection, bleeding, or other complications.

Sometimes bed rest and hydration—extra fluids given by mouth or through a tube inserted into a vein—are enough to stop contractions. You may also be given medications that stop contractions. These will be started in the hospital and any need to continue medication at home will be reviewed with you.

You may be able to go home if you are not really in preterm labor or if labor is stopped. Otherwise, you may need to stay in the hospital for a while. This depends upon what the health care provider's exam reveals and other factors.

Limit Your Activity

If you have had preterm labor, limits on activity may be prescribed. If you have a job that requires heavy lifting or standing a lot, it may require some changes. You may have to stop working. You may be advised to go on partial bed rest, which means you can get up, go to the bathroom, and have limited activity. You may be advised to stay off your feet and not do certain activities, such as climbing stairs. You may be confined to total bed rest.

For most women, having to limit your activity week after week is very hard. You may often feel moody, helpless, and depressed. Sometimes you may feel that the frustration and boredom just are not worth it, and you may be tempted to resume your activities.

If you must limit your activity, structure your life to help lessen your frustration. Do not be afraid to rely on others for support.

Because you will be less active, you may need to make changes in your diet so you take in fewer calories. High-fiber foods, such as fresh fruits and vegetables and whole grain products, and plenty of fluids will help you avoid constipation.

If bed rest is prescribed, plan your days to include a change into day clothes and tasks that you can do in bed, perhaps with a phone nearby. You may want to talk to your health care provider about exercises you can do in bed to improve your circulation.

Preterm Delivery

Sometimes preterm labor may be too advanced to be stopped, or there may be reasons that the baby is better off being born, even if it is early. These

✤ **It's A Fact!!**

Preterm labor, delivery, and care of the baby require care in a hospital with special facilities.

can include infection, high blood pressure, bleeding, or signs that the fetus may be having problems. Preterm babies may be delivered by cesarean birth, in which the baby is born through an incision made in the mother's abdomen and uterus. Some preterm babies are delivered vaginally.

Your Preterm Baby

Many preterm babies are tiny and fragile. Depending on how early the baby is born, he or she may need special medical care in order to breathe, eat, and keep warm. Preterm babies can have physical and mental disabilities that can be long-term. Babies born before 32 weeks of pregnancy are most at risk.

Preterm babies may not be ready to live on their own. They may be cared for in a neonatal intensive care unit (NICU) for weeks and sometimes months. Preterm babies are often kept in an incubator to keep them warm. They are cared for by specially trained nurses and other health care providers. Today, with special NICU care, even very early, tiny babies have a much better chance of survival than in the past. In spite of the best medical care, though, not all preterm babies survive.

Physical Features

Preterm babies are usually of low birth weight (weighing less than 5 and 1/2 pounds at birth). Babies born too early often have organs that are not developed enough to function properly. For instance, the lungs of a preterm baby are often not fully developed, and the newborn may have trouble getting enough air. This condition is called respiratory distress syndrome (RDS). Sometimes a woman in preterm labor is given drugs to reduce the risks to the baby. Other drugs could be given to the baby after birth to improve breathing. Your baby may be placed on a respirator to help with breathing. Apnea, or interrupted breathing, often occurs in preterm and low birth weight babies in the first days or weeks of life.

Your preterm baby may not look like what you expected. Most preterm babies are quite red and skinny because they have less fat under their skin and their blood vessels are close to the surface. After a few days, your preterm baby may develop jaundice, causing his or her skin to appear yellow. This condition is temporary.

A preterm baby may also have problems with swallowing. This means he or she may need to be fed through a tube. You may need to express or pump your breasts to provide breast milk to your baby.

Emotional Needs

Hospitals are often busy, crowded places. At first, you may feel that everyone else is taking care of your baby, and there is no place for you. You may wish for privacy. You may feel frightened and awkward. These are normal reactions to this new situation. Talk to the health care providers caring for your baby. They will help you with any questions you may have and advise you on how often you should visit the baby.

Your baby needs to hear your voice and to feel your touch. Contact with the baby is important for the parents, too. As soon as you can, talk to your baby. Stroke him or her in the incubator. After a while, you may be able to hold and cuddle your baby for longer periods of time and help with the baby's care.

Care At Home

If you have a preterm delivery, it is especially important for you to follow instructions about care for your new baby. Preterm babies usually require more health care provider visits in the first few months at home. This may include special eye and ear exams. You may have to give your baby special medicines, vitamins, or feeding supplements.

Some preterm babies can leave the hospital but need to take extra oxygen at home. You may need to watch for signs of breathing problems (wheezing, congestion). Sometimes monitors can be used to check the baby's breathing. You should be prepared to perform infant cardiopulmonary resuscitation (CPR) in case of an emergency. Depending on the size of your baby, a standard infant car seat may actually be dangerous to use. Discuss this with your health care provider.

Your preterm baby may be more irritable, more active, and more dependent on you than other children would be. Be patient and get support when you need it. There are many support services available to help you through this demanding time. The hospital staff can discuss this with you.

☞ Remember!!

Although the exact causes of preterm labor are not known, there are things you can do to improve your baby's chances of being born healthy. Regular prenatal care is an important first step in preventing preterm labor. Lead a healthy lifestyle, be alert to warning signs, and follow your health care provider's advice.

Chapter 34

Birth-Related Injuries

Birth injury is damage sustained during the birthing process, usually occurring during transit through the birth canal.

A difficult delivery, with the risk of injury to the fetus, may occur if the birth canal is too small or the fetus is too large (as sometimes occurs when the mother has diabetes). Injury is also more likely if the fetus is lying in an abnormal position before birth. Overall, the rate of birth injuries is much lower now than in previous decades.

Many newborns experience minor injuries from the birthing process, with swelling or bruising only in certain areas.

Head Injury: In most births, the head is the first part to enter the birth canal and experiences much of the pressure during the delivery. Swelling and bruising are not serious and resolve within a few days. Cephalohematoma is a bleeding injury in which a soft lump forms over the surface of one of the skull bones but below its thick fibrous covering. A cephalohematoma does not need treatment and disappears over weeks to months.

About This Chapter: Information in this chapter is from "Birth Injury," *The Merck Manual of Medical Information—Second Home Edition*, pp. 1494–1495, edited by Mark H. Beers. Copyright 2003 by Merck and Co., Inc., Whitehouse Station, NJ. Reprinted with permission. Merck Manuals are available free online at www.MerckManuals.com.

♣ It's A Fact!!
Common Birthmarks And Minor Skin Conditions In The Newborn

There are a number of skin conditions that are considered normal in the newborn. There may be bruises or marks from forceps on the newborn's face and scalp, or bruising of the feet following a breech delivery, all of which resolve within just a few days. Pink marks that are due to dilated capillaries under the skin may be seen on the forehead just above the nose, in the upper eyelids, or at the back of the neck (where it is called "stork-bite"). This type of birthmark fades as the infant grows but in some people remains as a faint mark that becomes brighter when the person becomes excited or upset. Some newborns have a few acne pimples, especially over the cheeks and forehead. These go away, and the only recommended action is to keep the skin clean and not to use creams or lotions.

Milia are tiny, pearly white cysts that are normally found over the nose and upper cheeks. Milia become smaller or disappear over a period of weeks. Similar white cysts are sometimes found on the gums or in the midline of the roof of the mouth (Epstein pearls) and are also of no consequence.

Mongolian spots are bluish gray flat areas that usually occur over the lower back or buttocks. At first glance, they appear to be bruises but are not. They are usually seen in black or Asian newborns and are of no consequence.

A "strawberry hemangioma" is a common birthmark. It is a flat, slightly pink or red area anywhere on the skin. Over a period of weeks, it becomes darker red and also becomes raised up over the surface of the skin, appearing much as a strawberry. After several years, strawberry hemangiomas shrink and become fainter, so that by the time the child reaches school age, most are no longer visible. For this reason, surgery is not needed.

Very rarely, one of the bones of the skull may fracture. Unless the fracture forms an indentation (depressed fracture), it heals rapidly without treatment.

Nerve Injury: Rarely, nerve injuries may occur. Pressure to the facial nerves caused by forceps can result in weakness of the muscles on one side of the face. This injury is evident when the newborn cries and the face appears asymmetric. No treatment is needed, and the newborn usually recovers within a few weeks.

In a difficult delivery of a large infant, some of the larger nerves to one or both of the newborn's arms can be stretched and injured. Weakness (paralysis) of the newborn's arm or hand results. Occasionally, the nerve going to the diaphragm (the muscle that separates the organs of the chest from those of the abdomen) is damaged, resulting in paralysis of the diaphragm on the same side. In this case, the newborn may have difficulty breathing. Injury of the nerves to the newborn's arm and diaphragm usually resolves completely within a few weeks. Extreme movements at the shoulder should be avoided to allow the nerves to heal. Very rarely, the arm and possibly the diaphragm remain weak after several months. In this case, surgery may be needed to reattach torn nerves.

Injuries to the spinal cord due to overstretching during delivery are extremely rare. These injuries can result in paralysis below where the injury occurred. Damage to the spinal cord is often permanent.

Bone Injury: Rarely, bones may be broken (fractured) during a difficult delivery. A fracture of the collarbone is most common. Fractures of bones in the newborn are splinted and almost always heal completely and rapidly.

Chapter 35

Miscarriage And Stillbirth

Losing a pregnancy can be heartbreaking. And for many expectant couples, the fear of having a miscarriage can be consuming, even edging out the excitement about being pregnant.

In most cases, a miscarriage cannot be prevented because it is the result of a random genetic or chromosomal change that occurs during conception or during early fetal development. That said, certain factors—such as age, smoking, drinking, and a history of miscarriage—put a woman at a higher risk for losing a pregnancy. But you can do many things to increase the chances that you and your baby will be healthy throughout the pregnancy.

What Is A Miscarriage?

A miscarriage is the spontaneous abortion of an embryo or fetus before it's developed enough to survive. This can happen even before a woman is aware that she is pregnant.

A miscarriage usually occurs in the first three months of pregnancy, before 20 weeks' gestation. A small fraction of miscarriages—less than 1% of them—are called stillbirths, as they occur after 20 weeks of gestation.

About This Chapter: This information, "Miscarriages," was provided by KidsHealth, one of the largest resources online for medically reviewed health information written for parents, kids, and teens. For more articles like this one, visit www.KidsHealth.org, or www.TeensHealth.org. © 2005 The Nemours Foundation.

Symptoms Of A Miscarriage

Many women don't even know that they've had a miscarriage, thinking that it's just a particularly heavy menstrual flow.

Some women experience cramping, spotting, abdominal pain, fever, weakness, vomiting, or back pain. Spotting is not always a sign of a miscarriage; many women normally experience it early on in pregnancy. But just to be safe, if you have spotting or any of these other symptoms anytime during your pregnancy, it's a good idea to talk with your doctor.

♣ **It's A Fact!!**

Unfortunately, miscarriages are fairly common. On average, one in five pregnancies will end in a miscarriage—and some research shows that there are up to 800,000 miscarriages a year in the United States.

If you have had a miscarriage, your doctor may use a number of terms to explain what has happened. Your doctor may say you have a blighted ovum, which is a miscarriage that has occurred so early that no clearly defined fetal tissues have formed. An inevitable miscarriage is bleeding and cramping during the early stages of a pregnancy, signs that the cervix may be opening. An incomplete miscarriage is when the body does not expel all the elements of the pregnancy. A missed miscarriage is when the body does not discharge the fetus, the placenta, or other elements for several weeks—this might occur when the woman has neither menstrual periods nor any signs of pregnancy. A recurrent abortion is when a woman miscarries three or more consecutive times.

Stillbirths

A stillbirth, the death of a baby after the 20th week of pregnancy, can occur before delivery or as a result of complications of labor or delivery. It is very rare and occurs in less than 1% of all births. A stillbirth also is sometimes referred to as intrauterine fetal death or antenatal death.

The first and most common sign of a stillbirth is lack of movement in the baby as the due date approaches. This might be accompanied by persistent cramping or stabbing pains in the pelvis, back, or lower abdomen, or vaginal bleeding. If you experience any of these symptoms, talk to your doctor.

Your doctor can listen for the fetal heartbeat with a stethoscope, use Doppler ultrasound to detect the heartbeat, or give you an electronic fetal non-stress test, which involves lying on your back with electronic monitors attached to your abdomen. The monitors record the baby's heart rate, movements, and contractions of the uterus.

Why Do Miscarriages And Stillbirths Happen?

The most common cause of pregnancy loss is a random chromosome abnormality that occurs during fertilization. For fertilization to occur, the chromosomes in the nucleus of both the egg and the sperm need to join into 23 pairs (46 total chromosomes). Sometimes this pairing does not happen correctly and that can impede the development of the fetus.

Other factors that could contribute to a miscarriage include the following:

♣ **It's A Fact!!**

There is no way to predict when stillbirth will happen or who will have one, and the cause of about one-third of all stillbirths remains unknown.

- fertilization late after ovulation

- low or high levels of the thyroid hormone

- uncontrolled diabetes

- exposure to environmental and workplace hazards, such as radiation or toxic agents

- uterine abnormalities

- incompetent cervix, or when the cervix begins to open (dilate) and thin (efface) before the pregnancy has reached term

- certain medications (mostly prescription), such as the acne drug Accutane

Certain behaviors also increase the risk of a miscarriage. Smoking, for example, puts nicotine and other chemicals into the bloodstream that cause the blood vessels in the placenta to spasm, which decreases the blood flow to the uterus. Smokers also have a lower level of oxygen in their blood, which means the fetus gets less oxygen. Alcohol and illegal drugs have been proved to lead to miscarriages. There is no evidence that stress or sexual activity contributes to miscarriage.

Some of the common causes of a stillbirth include the following:

- preeclampsia and eclampsia, disorders of late pregnancy that involve high blood pressure, fluid retention, and protein in the urine

- uncontrolled diabetes

- abnormalities in the fetus caused by infectious diseases—such as syphilis, toxoplasmosis, German measles, rubella, and influenza—or by bacterial infections like listeriosis

- severe birth defects (responsible for about 20% of stillbirths), including spina bifida

- post maturity—a condition in which the pregnancy has lasted 41 weeks or longer

- chronic high blood pressure, lupus, heart, or thyroid disease

What Will Happen After A Miscarriage Or Stillbirth?

If you have miscarried, your doctor will do a pelvic exam and an ultrasound test to confirm the miscarriage. If the uterus is clear of any fetal tissue, then there won't be any more treatment. But if the uterus still contains the fetus or portions of the fetus, the doctor will dilate the cervix to perform a dilation and curettage (D&C)—a scraping of the uterine lining—or a dilation and extraction (D&E)—a suction of the uterus to remove fetal or placental tissue. You may have spotting or mild cramping after these procedures, which are done under local or general anesthesia so there is no immediate pain.

If it is determined that your baby has died in utero after the 20th week, the doctor might decide to induce labor and delivery. After the delivery, the doctor will examine the baby and the placenta to help determine the cause of death if it's still unknown.

If you've had several miscarriages, you may want to be evaluated to see if any anatomic, genetic, or hormonal abnormalities are contributing to the miscarriages.

Can Miscarriages Or Stillbirths Be Prevented?

Although miscarriage and stillbirths usually can't be prevented, there are precautions you can take to increase your chances of having a healthy pregnancy:

- Maintain a proper diet loaded with folic acid and calcium.

- Exercise after you've gotten your doctor's OK.

- Avoid drugs and alcohol.

- Avoid deli meats and soft cheeses such as feta and other foods that could carry listeriosis.

- Limit caffeine drinks to no more than one to two cups a day.

- Stop smoking.

- Talk to your doctor about all medications you're currently taking. Unless your doctor indicates otherwise, many prescription and over-the-counter medicines should be avoided during pregnancy.

- Avoid abdominal trauma.

- Get immunized against communicable disease and know your family medical and genetic history.

Part Five

Childbirth: Are You Prepared?

Chapter 36

Nine Months: How Your Baby Grows

First Month

About five to seven days after a sperm fertilizes an egg, the egg attaches to the lining of the uterus. This process is called implantation. The fertilized egg then begins to grow in the uterus, doubling in size every day. At this stage of development the baby is called an embryo.

Shortly after implantation, the placenta and umbilical cord begin to form. The placenta and umbilical cord provide nourishment and oxygen to the baby and carry away the baby's wastes. The baby is enclosed in a sac of fluid, called the amniotic sac, to protect the baby from bumps and pressure.

In another week, the baby has a spinal cord. A few days later, five to eight bones of the spinal column (vertebrae) are in place. Nerve development is beginning. By the end of the first six weeks of pregnancy, the baby has a head and trunk.

The embryo becomes three layers around the fifth week. The outer layer consists of the brain, nerves, and skin. The middle layer becomes the bones, muscles, blood vessels, heart, and sex organs. The inner layer holds the

About This Chapter: Information in this chapter is excerpted from "The Growth and Development of Your Baby." Reprinted with permission from the University of Michigan Health System, www.med.umich.edu. Copyright © 2005 Regents of the University of Michigan.

stomach, liver, intestines, lungs, and urinary tract. The eyes and other features begin to form, as do tiny buds that will be the arms and legs. The heart also forms, and it begins to beat on the 25th day after conception (five to six weeks after the last menstrual period). However, it is impossible to hear the heart beating at this time.

By the end of six weeks, the baby is about 1/2 inch long and weighs a fraction of an ounce.

Second Month

This month is especially critical in the development of the baby. Any disturbance from drugs, viruses, or environmental factors, such as pesticides, may cause birth defects.

The baby's development is very rapid during the second month. By the end of the second month, all of the baby's major body organs and body systems, including the brain, lungs, liver, and stomach, have begun to develop. The first bone cells appear during this time. Eyelids form and grow but remain sealed shut. The inner ear is forming. Ankles, toes, wrists, fingers, and sexual organs are developing.

At the end of the second month of pregnancy, the baby looks like a tiny human infant. If it is a boy, the penis will begin to appear. The baby is a little over one inch long and still weighs less than one ounce. From now on the baby is called a fetus.

Third Month

The baby will be completely formed by the end of the third month. The baby may have begun moving its hands, legs, and head, and opening and closing its mouth, but he or she is still too small for the mother to feel this movement.

The fingers and toes are now more distinct and have soft nails. The baby's hands are more developed than the feet, and the arms are longer than the legs. The baby's head is quite large compared to the rest of its body. Hair may have started to form on the head. Tooth buds have formed under the baby's gums. Vocal cords develop around the 13th week of pregnancy.

The baby's heart has four chambers and beats at 120 to 160 beats per minute. Kidneys are now developed and start draining urine into the bladder. Intestines have formed outside of the baby (on the umbilical cord) because they cannot fit inside the baby. By the end of this month, the umbilical cord, which carries nutrients to the baby and takes wastes away, will be fully formed.

At the end of the third month, the baby will weigh just over one ounce and will be about four inches long.

Fourth Month

The baby's skin is pink and somewhat transparent. Eyebrows and eyelashes begin to appear in this month. Buds on the side of the head begin to form into the outer ear. The baby's face continues to develop. The tail has disappeared from the fetus and the head makes up about half of the baby's size. The baby's neck is long enough to lift the head from the body.

The baby moves, kicks, sleeps, wakes, swallows, and passes urine. The mother may start to feel a slight sensation in her lower abdomen (called quickening). This feels like bubbles or fluttering. When the mother feels the baby's movement, she should write down the date and tell her health care provider. This helps determine when the baby is due.

By the end of the fourth month, the baby will be eight to ten inches long and will weigh about six ounces.

Fifth Month

This is a period of tremendous growth for the baby. The internal organs are maturing. The baby's fingernails have grown to the tips of the fingers. Fat is now being stored beneath the baby's skin. The baby is also growing muscle and is getting stronger every day. The blood cells take over for the liver the job of producing blood. The baby's gall bladder will become functional, producing bile that is necessary for digestion. Milk teeth will begin forming under the baby's gums. Body hair, including eyebrows and eyelashes, are starting to grow.

✎ What's It Mean?

Ovaries: Part of a woman's reproductive system, the ovaries produce her eggs. Each month, through the process called ovulation, the ovaries release eggs into the fallopian tubes, where they travel to the uterus, or womb. If a man's sperm fertilizes an egg, a woman becomes pregnant and the egg grows and develops inside the uterus. If the egg is not fertilized, the egg and the lining of the uterus are shed during a woman's monthly menstrual period. [1]

Placenta: During pregnancy, a temporary organ joining the mother and fetus. The placenta transfers oxygen and nutrients from the mother to the fetus and permits the release of carbon dioxide and waste products from the fetus. The placenta is expelled during the birth process with the fetal membranes. [1]

Scrotum: In males, the external sac that contains the testicles. [2]

Sperm: The male reproductive cell, formed in the testicle. A sperm unites with an egg to form an embryo. [2]

Testicles (Testes): The male sex gland. There is a pair of testes behind the penis in a pouch of skin called the scrotum. The testes make and store sperm and make the male hormone testosterone. [1]

Umbilical Cord: Connected to the placenta and provides the transfer of nutrients and waste between the woman and the fetus. [1]

Uterus: A woman's womb, or the hollow, pear-shaped organ located in a woman's lower abdomen between the bladder and the rectum. [1]

Source: [1] "NWHIC Web Site Glossary," National Women's Health Information Center, U.S. Department of Health and Human Services, cited August 2006. [2] "Dictionary of Cancer Terms," National Cancer Institute, U.S. National Institutes of Health; cited August 2006.

The baby sleeps and wakes at regular intervals. The mother will find that the baby is much more active now. He or she turns from side to side and head over heels. The baby may suck its thumb.

At the end of the fifth month, the baby will be about 10 to 12 inches long and will weigh about one pound.

Sixth Month

This month continues to be a period of rapid growth. The baby's skin is wrinkled and red. It is covered with lanugo (fine, soft hair) and vernix (a substance consisting of oil, sloughed skin cells, and lanugo). Real hair and toenails are beginning to grow. The baby's brain is developing rapidly. Fatty sheaths, which transmit electrical impulses along nerves, are forming. Meconium, the baby's first stool, is developing. A special type of fat (brown fat), which keeps the baby warm at birth, is forming. Baby girls will develop eggs in their ovaries during this month. The baby's bones are becoming solid.

The baby is almost fully formed and looks like a miniature human. However, because the lungs are not well developed and the baby is still very small, a baby cannot usually live outside the uterus at this stage without highly specialized care.

By the end of the sixth month, the baby will be around 11 to 14 inches long and will weigh about 1 to 1 1/2 pounds.

Seventh Month

The baby is continuing to grow and develop. The baby's eyes can now open and close and can sense light changes. The lanugo is starting to disappear from the baby's face. The baby's hearing is getting better. He or she can now hear the outside world quite well over the sound of your heartbeat. The baby exercises by kicking and stretching. He or she can also make grasping motions and likes to suck its thumb.

By the end of this month, the baby will be approximately 15 inches long and weigh about 2 or 2 1/2 pounds. If the baby was born now, its chances of survival are better than last month.

Eighth Month

The baby's body continues to grow quickly. The bones are getting stronger, limbs are fatter, and the skin has a healthy glow. The brain is now forming its different regions. The brain and nerves are directing bodily functions. Taste buds are developing. The baby may now hiccup, cry, taste sweet and sour, and respond to pain, light, and sound. If the baby is a boy, his testicles have dropped from his abdomen, where they will then descend into his scrotum.

The baby will be about 16 to 18 inches long and will weigh about 4 pounds at the end of this month.

Ninth Month

The baby is now gaining about a 1/2 pound each week. The baby is getting fatter and its skin is less rumpled. He or she is getting ready for birth and is settling into the fetal position with its head down against the birth canal, its legs tucked up to its chest, and its knees against its nose.

The mother's antibodies to disease are beginning to flow rapidly through the placenta. The rapid flow of blood through the umbilical cord keeps it taut, which prevents tangles.

The baby is beginning to develop sleeping patterns. The baby will continue to kick and punch, although it will move lower in the mother's abdomen to under her pelvis (this is a process called "lightening"). The mother will also feel the baby roll around as it gets too cramped inside the uterus for much movement. The baby's lungs are now mature and the baby will have a great chance of survival if born a little early. The bones of the baby's head are soft and flexible to ease the process of delivery through the birth canal.

The baby is now about 20 inches long and weighs approximately 6 to 9 pounds. The baby may be born anytime between the 37th and 42nd week of pregnancy. Only 5 percent of babies are born on their due date.

Chapter 37

Preparing In Advance For Your Baby's Arrival: Items Your Baby Will Need

During your pregnancy, you have so many decisions to make and so much to prepare before your new baby is born. You may want to begin purchasing clothing, a car seat, and furniture for the baby. Do not forget about all the items your new baby will need on a daily basis such as diapers, washcloths, bottles, burp cloths, and more. If you are having a baby shower, your friends and family may also ask you what items they can help you with. There are so many baby items and different brands to choose from, that it may be helpful to get some expert advice so that you will not be stressed about these decisions.

What The Baby Will Need At The Hospital

• undershirt

• an outfit such as a stretch suit, nightgown, or sweater set

• a pair of socks or booties

• receiving blanket, cap and heavier blanket or bunting (if the weather is cold)

• diapers and wipes (some hospitals provide an initial supply of these)

About This Chapter: Information in this chapter is from "Baby Shopping List," National Women's Health Information Center, U.S. Department of Health and Human Services, January 2006.

- safety pins or Velcro attaching strips, and rubber or nylon pants (if you are using cloth diapers)

- infant car seat

- diaper bag

Safety Items For The Home

- nightlights or soft lighting

- baby monitor

- baby nail clippers/scissors manicure set

Things You Will Need To Transport The Baby

- car seat

- stroller

- backpacks and soft carriers

- diaper

Items For The Baby's Room

- crib and crib linens

- playpen or portable crib

- changing table

- dresser

- glider or rocking chair

- clothes hamper

✔ Quick Tip

Talk to other new moms about the items they purchased for their babies and the brands that they recommend.

Source: The National Women's Health
Information Center.

♣ It's A Fact!!
Guidelines For Buying Children's Sleepwear

The U.S. Consumer Product Safety Commission sets national safety standards for children's sleepwear flammability. These standards are designed to protect children from burn injuries if they come in contact with an open flame such as a match or stove burner. Under amended federal safety rules, garments sold as children's sleepwear for sizes larger than nine months must be one of the following:

Flame Resistant: Flame resistant garments do not continue burning when removed from an ignition source. An example would be inherently flame resistant polyesters that do not require chemical treatment.

Or

Snug Fitting: Snug fitting garments need not be flame resistant because they are made to fit closely against a child's body. Snug-fitting sleepwear does not ignite easily; and, even if ignited, does not burn readily because there is little oxygen to feed a fire.

The rules for flame resistance or snug fit do not apply to sleepwear for sizes nine months and under because infants that wear these sizes are insufficiently mobile to expose themselves to an open flame.

Children should never be put to sleep in T-shirts, sweats, or other oversized, loose-fitting cotton or cotton-blend garments. These garments can catch fire easily and are associated with 200 to 300 emergency room-treated burn injuries to children annually.

Most manufacturers are using hangtags on their snug-fitting sleepwear to let consumers know that the product meets federal safety standards. The hangtags remind consumers that a snug fit or flame resistance is necessary for safety.

Source: Consumer Product Safety Commission (www.cpsc.gov); cited August 2006.

Suggested Items For Your Home

- diapers
- receiving blankets
- clothing
- breast pump (if you plan to breastfeed)
- bottles (be sure to get the correct size of nipples such as preemie or newborn)
- rectal or digital ear thermometer
- bathtub
- washcloths and baby wipes
- diaper rash ointment and/or petroleum jelly
- hooded towels
- diaper disposal system (good to have but not necessary)
- burp cloths and waterproof lap pads
- bulb syringe (for suctioning baby's nasal passages if necessary)

Things You Will Need As The Baby Gets Older

- outlet protectors
- toys
- books
- walker
- high chair
- gates

Chapter 38

Birthing Classes

If you are having a child for the first time, it is easy to feel overwhelmed by questions, fears, and just not knowing what to expect. Many new parents find that birthing classes can really help calm their worries and answer many questions.

These classes cover all kinds of issues surrounding childbirth including breathing techniques, pain management, vaginal labor, and cesarean labor. They can help prepare you for many aspects of childbirth: for the changes that pregnancy brings, for labor and delivery, and for parenting once your baby is born.

Typically, new parents take birthing classes around the third trimester of the pregnancy, when the mother is about six months pregnant. But there are a variety of different kinds of classes, which begin both sooner and later than that. It's a good idea to talk with your doctor about the different kinds of classes that are offered in your community.

Benefits Of Taking A Childbirth Class

A childbirth class can provide you with a great forum to ask lots of questions and can help you make informed decisions about the key issues

About This Chapter: This information was provided by KidsHealth, one of the largest resources online for medically reviewed health information written for parents, kids, and teens. For more articles like this one, visit www.KidsHealth.org, or www.TeensHealth.org. © 2005 The Nemours Foundation.

surrounding your baby's birth. Some of the information you can find out from a birthing class includes the following:

- how your baby is developing

- healthy developments in your pregnancy

- warning signs that something is wrong

- how to make your pregnancy, labor, and delivery more comfortable

- breathing and relaxation techniques

- how to write a birth plan

- how to tell when you are in labor

- pain relief options during labor

- the role of the coach or labor partner

Many classes also address what to expect after the baby is born, including breastfeeding, baby care, and dealing with the emotional changes of new parenthood.

You might also find support from other expectant couples at a childbirth class. Who would better understand the ups and downs of pregnancy than couples who are going through them, too? Many people find friends in their childbirth class who last long past the birth of their child.

If your birth coach is also the baby's father, taking a class together can mean his increased involvement in the pregnancy. Like the mother, the father can also benefit from knowing what to expect when the mother goes into labor—and how to assist in that process. Some classes have one session just for fathers, where men can discuss their own concerns about pregnancy and birth. There are also classes geared just for new fathers. Some classes even offer a special session for new grandparents, which is a great way to get them involved in the process and to make sure they're up on the latest in baby care techniques and safety.

Of course, some people get more out of childbirth classes than others do. But even if you find the techniques you're taught don't work for you when you finally go into labor, you may get other benefits from the class. The common goal of all birthing classes is to provide you with the knowledge and confidence you need to give birth and make informed decisions. This includes reducing your anxiety about the birth experience, as well as providing you with a variety of coping techniques to aid in pain management. Remember that the ultimate goal is to have a healthy mom and healthy baby.

What Types Of Classes Are Available?

The Lamaze technique is the most widely used method in the United States. The Lamaze philosophy holds that birth is a normal, natural, and healthy process and that women should be empowered through education and support to approach it with confidence. The goal of Lamaze is to explore all the ways women can find strength and comfort during labor and birth. Classes focus on relaxation techniques, but they also encourage the mother to condition her body's response to pain through training and practice (this is called psychoprophylaxis). This conditioning is meant to teach expectant mothers constructive responses to the pain and stress of labor (for example, controlled breathing patterns) as opposed to counterproductive responses (such as holding the breath or tensing up). Other techniques, such as distraction (a woman might be encouraged to focus on a special object from home or a photo, for example) or massage by a supportive coach, are also used to decrease a woman's perception of pain.

Lamaze courses don't advocate for or against the use of drugs and routine medical interventions during labor and delivery, but instead educate mothers about their options so they can make informed decisions when the time comes.

The Bradley method (also called "Husband-Coached Birth") places an emphasis on a natural approach to birth and on the active participation of the baby's father as the birth coach. A major goal of this method is the avoidance of medications unless absolutely necessary.

Other topics stressed include the importance of good nutrition and exercise during pregnancy, relaxation techniques (such as deep breathing and concentration on body signals) as a method of coping with labor, and the empowerment of parents to trust their instincts and become active, informed participants in the birth process. The course is traditionally offered in 12 sessions.

Although Bradley emphasizes a birth experience without pain medication, the classes do prepare parents for unexpected complications or situations, like emergency cesarean sections. After the birth, immediate breast-feeding and constant contact between parents and baby is stressed. Bradley is the method of choice for many women who give birth at home or in other nonhospital settings.

There are several other types of birthing classes available. Some include information from the two previously mentioned techniques, and some are offshoots that explore one particular area. Two options that might be available in your area are active birth classes that teach yoga techniques to prepare for labor and "hypnobirthing" courses, which use hypnosis as a relaxation technique.

When Should I Start Taking A Birthing Class?

In addition to offering many techniques and curricula, birthing classes also vary greatly in terms of duration. You'll find classes that begin during the first trimester and focus on all the changes that pregnancy brings; 5- to 8-week courses offered late in pregnancy aimed at educating parents mostly about labor, delivery, and postpartum issues; and one-time-only refresher courses for repeat parents. Most parents opt for a course that meets about six or seven times in the last trimester for 1 1/2 to 2 hours per session, or for full-day versions that take place over one or two weekends. What's important to remember is that a variety of options are often offered, so be sure and find one that fits your needs.

Choosing A Birthing Class

The type of class that's right for you depends on your personality and beliefs, as well as those of your labor partner. There is no one correct method. If you're the kind of person who likes to share and is eager to meet people, you might like a smaller, more intimate class designed for couples to swap stories and support each other. If you don't like the idea of sharing in a small group, you might want a larger class, where the teacher does most of the talking.

Of course, the community you live in may limit your choices—expectant parents in rural areas often have fewer choices than those in large cities. You may find childbirth classes offered by the following:

- hospitals

- private teachers

- health care providers (through their practices)

- community health organizations

- midwives

- national childbirth education organizations

- videos and DVDs

Before you sign up for a class, it's a good idea to ask what the curriculum includes and what philosophy it is based upon. You can also request to see the course outline. A good class will cover a range of topics and prepare you for the many possible scenarios of labor and delivery. Classes should include information about vaginal births and cesarean sections; natural childbirth techniques as well as the use of pain medication during labor; tips on pre- and postnatal care; and postpartum adjustment.

If something you wanted or expected to see isn't included in the outline, ask about it—if your teacher doesn't seem flexible or his or her philosophy doesn't match yours, you may want to look elsewhere.

You should also feel free to contact the teacher or childbirth class coordinator with questions, such as the following:

- What's your background and how were you trained?

- Do you have certification from a nationally recognized organization?

- What is your philosophy? Do you teach a particular method?

- How does the class time break down between lecture, discussion, and practicing techniques?

- How many people are in the class?

Finding A Birthing Class

✔ Quick Tip

Whatever course or method you choose, you'll want to begin exploring your options early—some classes fill up well in advance of the start date.

There are a variety of ways you can find out about your birthing class options. A good place to start is with your obstetrician, family doctor, or midwife, followed by friends or acquaintances who have had babies in your area. Your local hospital or birthing center should also be able to provide you with a list of classes.

You can also contact national organizations that certify childbirth educators. The International Childbirth Education Association supports families and trains childbirth educators—you can contact them to find out what certified courses are offered in your area. Lamaze International can give you information on where the Lamaze technique is taught in your area; for information on the Bradley method, contact the American Academy of Husband-Coached Childbirth.

Whether it's a healthier pregnancy, increased knowledge, reduced anxiety, or a greater closeness with your labor partner, there are many benefits to taking a birthing class.

Chapter 39

Birth Plans

The term birth plan can actually be misleading—it's less an exact plan than a list of preferences. In fact, the best thing about a birth plan isn't that it allows you and your partner to determine exactly how the birth of your child will occur—because labor involves so many variables, you can't predict exactly what will happen. A birth plan does, however, help you to realize what's most important to you in the birth of your baby.

While completing a birth plan, you'll be learning about, exploring, and understanding your labor and birthing options well before the birth of your child. Not only will this improve your communication with the people who'll be helping during your delivery, it also means you won't have to explain your preferences right at the moment when you're least in the mood for conversation—during labor itself.

What Questions Does A Birth Plan Answer?

A birth plan typically covers three major areas.

About This Chapter: Information in this chapter was provided by KidsHealth, one of the largest resources online for medically reviewed health information written for parents, kids, and teens. For more articles like this one, visit www.KidsHealth.org, or www.TeensHealth.org. © 2004 The Nemours Foundation.

What Are Your Wishes During A Normal Labor And Delivery?

These range from how you'll handle pain relief to enemas and fetal monitoring. Think about the environment in which you want to have your baby, who you want to have there, and what birthing positions you plan to use.

How Do You Want Your Baby To Be Treated Immediately After And For The First Few Days After Birth?

Do you want the baby's cord to be cut by your partner? Should your baby be placed on your stomach immediately after birth? Do you want to feed the baby immediately? Will you breastfeed or bottle-feed? Where will the baby sleep—next to you or in the nursery? Hospitals have widely varying policies for the care of newborns—if you choose to have your baby in a hospital, you'll want to know what these are and whether they match your wishes.

What Do You Want To Happen In The Case Of Unexpected Events?

No one wants to think about something going wrong, but if it does, it's better to be prepared than to have to make snap decisions when you're upset. Given the number of women who have cesarean sections (C-sections), your birth plan should probably cover your wishes in the event that your labor takes an unexpected turn. You might also want to think about other possible complications, such as premature birth.

Factors To Consider

Before you make decisions about each of your birthing options, you'll want to talk with your health care provider and tour the hospital or birthing center where you plan to have your baby.

> ### ♣ It's A Fact!!
>
> A birth plan isn't a binding agreement—it's just a guideline. Your doctor or health care provider should know, from having seen you throughout the pregnancy, what you do and don't want. But a well thought-out birth plan is your best guarantee that the delivery of your child will go according to your wishes.

You may find that your obstetrician, nurse-midwife, or the facility where they admit patients already has birth plan forms that you can fill out. If this is the case, you can use the form as a guideline for asking questions about how women in their care are routinely treated. If their responses don't meet your expectations of how you'd like to be treated, you may want to switch health care providers, if at all possible. Also, finding out what normally happens allows you to leave information out of your birth plan, if you know your wishes are going to be met as part of routine care.

And it's important to be flexible—if you know one aspect of your birthing plan won't be met, be sure to weigh that aspect against your other wishes. If your options are limited because of insurance, cost, or geography, focus on one or two areas that are really important to you. In the areas where your thinking doesn't agree with that of your doctor or nurse-midwife, ask why he or she usually does things a certain way and listen to his or her answers before you make up your mind.

Finally, you should find out if there are things about your pregnancy that might prevent certain choices. For example, if your pregnancy is considered high risk because of your age, health, or problems during previous pregnancies, your health care provider may advise against some of your birthing wishes. You'll want to discuss, and consider, this information when thinking about your options.

What Are Your Birthing Options?

In creating your plan, you're likely to have choices in the following areas.

Where To Have The Baby

Most women still give birth in the hospital. However, most women are no longer confined to a cold, sterile maternity ward. Find out if your hospital practices family-centered care. This usually means the patient rooms will have a door, furnishings, a private bathroom, and enough space to accommodate a family, including the baby's crib and supplies.

Additionally, many hospitals now offer birthing rooms that allow a woman to stay in the same bed for labor, delivery, and sometimes, postpartum care (care after the birth). These rooms are fully equipped for uncomplicated deliveries. They're often attractive and have gentle lighting.

But some women believe that the most comfortable environment is their own home. Advocates of home birth believe that labor and delivery can and should occur at home, but they also stress that a certified nurse-midwife or doctor should attend the birth.

☞ **Remember!!**

An important thing to remember about home birth is that if something goes wrong, you don't have the amenities and technology of a hospital.

For women with low-risk pregnancies who want something in between the hospital and home, birthing centers are a good option. These provide a more homey, relaxed environment with many of the medical amenities of a hospital.

Who Will Assist At The Birth

Most women choose an obstetrician (OB/GYN), a specialist who's trained to handle pregnancies (including those with complications), labor, and delivery. If your pregnancy is considered high risk, you may be referred to an obstetrician who sub specializes in perinatology (the care and treatment of the expectant mother and baby five months before and one month after the birth).

Another medical choice is a family practitioner who has had training and has maintained expertise in managing non-high-risk pregnancies and deliveries. In some areas of the United States, especially rural areas where obstetricians are less available, family practitioners handle most of the deliveries. One special benefit of choosing a family practitioner is that, as your family doctor, he or she can continue to treat both you and your baby after birth.

And doctors aren't the only health care providers a pregnant woman can choose to deliver her baby. You might decide that you want your delivery to be performed by a certified nurse-midwife, a health professional who's medically trained and licensed to handle low-risk births and whose philosophy emphasizes educating expectant parents about the natural aspects of childbirth.

Increasing numbers of women are choosing to have a doula, or birth assistant, present in addition to the medical personnel. This is someone who's trained in childbirth and is there to provide support to the mother. The doula meets with the mother before the birth and also helps to communicate her wishes to the medical staff, should it be necessary.

Your birth plan can also indicate who else you'd like to have with you before, during, and immediately after the birth. In a routine birth, this may be your partner, your other children, a friend, or other family member. You can also make it clear at what points you want no one to be there but your partner.

Atmosphere During Labor And Delivery

Many hospitals and birthing centers now allow women to make some choices about the atmosphere in which they give birth. Do you want music and low lighting? How about the freedom to walk around during labor? Is a hot tub something you'd like access to? Do you plan to eat or drink during labor? You might be able to request things that may make you the most comfortable—from what clothes you'll wear to whether you'll have a VCR or DVD player in your room.

Procedures During Labor

Hospitals used to perform the same procedures on all women in labor, but many now show increased flexibility in how they handle their patients. Some examples include the following:

- **Enemas:** Used to clean out the bowels, enemas used to be routinely administered when women were admitted. Now, you may choose to give yourself an enema or to skip it entirely.

- **Induction of labor:** Years ago, some doctors routinely induced labor. This is no longer done, unless there's a true medical need for it. Labor is allowed to take its natural course, with less medical intervention, in most hospital settings today.

- **Shaving the pubic area:** Once routine, shaving is no longer done unless a woman requests it.

Other procedures that you can include in your birth plan are requests about fetal monitoring, what types of birthing equipment you'd like in the room, and whether you have internal exams during labor.

Pain Management

This is important for most women and is certainly something you have a lot of control over. It's also something you'll want to discuss carefully with your health care provider. Many women change their minds about pain relief during labor only to discover that they're too far along in their labor to do anything about it. You'll also want to be aware of the alternate forms of pain relief, including massage, relaxation, breathing, hot tubs, sedatives, and tranquilizers. Know your options and make your wishes known to your health provider.

Position During Delivery

There are a variety of positions you can try during labor, including the classic semi-recline with the feet in stirrups that you've seen in the movies. Other choices include lying on your side, squatting, standing, or simply using whatever stance feels right at the time.

Episiotomies

When necessary, doctors perform episiotomies (when the perineum—the area of skin between the vagina and the anus—is cut to ease the delivery). You may have one if you risk tearing or in the case of a medical emergency.

Assisted Birth

If the baby becomes stuck in the birth canal, an assisted birth (i.e., using forceps or vacuum extraction) may be necessary. Find out what your doctor is most experienced with—that's probably your best choice.

Cesarean Section (C-Section)

You may not want to think about this, but if you have to have a cesarean, you'll need to consider a few things. Do you want your partner to be present, if possible? If you have a choice, would you like to be conscious or unconscious? What about viewing the birth—do you want to see the baby coming out?

Post-Birth

There are many decisions to make about the time immediately after birth, including the following:

• Would your partner like to cut the umbilical cord?

• Does your partner want to hold the baby when the baby emerges?

- Do you want immediate contact with the baby, or would you like the baby to be cleaned off first?

- How would you like to handle the delivery of the placenta? Would you like to keep the placenta?

- Do you want to feed the baby right away?

Communicating Your Wishes

Birth plans are relatively new inventions, and your doctor or nurse-midwife may not be completely comfortable with them. For this reason, make sure you communicate firmly and clearly that you intend to create a birth plan.

Give your health care provider your reasons for doing so—not because you don't trust him or her, but to help ensure cooperation and to cover the possibilities if something should go wrong. If your caregiver seems offended or is resistant to the idea of a birth plan, you may want to reconsider whether he or she is the right caregiver for you.

Once you've made your birth plan, schedule a time to go over it with your doctor or nurse-midwife. Find out and discuss where you agree or disagree. A few weeks before your due date, you might even want to consider going to the

---

✔ Quick Tip

Think about the language of your plan. You can use many online resources to create one or you can make one yourself. Here are some tips:

- Make your birth plan read like a list of requests or best-case scenarios, not like a set of demands. Phrases such as "I would prefer" and "if medically necessary" will help your health care provider and caregivers know that you understand that they might have to alter the plan.

- Think about the other personnel who'll be using it—hospital staffers may feel more comfortable if you call it your "birth preferences" rather than your "birth plan," which may seem as though you're trying to tell them how to do their jobs.

- Try to be positive ("We hope to") as opposed to negative ("Under no circumstances").

delivery area of the hospital or birth center where you plan to have your baby and share your plan with the staff there at a time when they aren't overly busy.

Strive to keep the plan as simple as possible—preferably less than two pages—and list your wishes in order of importance. Focusing on your priorities will help ensure that the most important of your wishes are met.

You may also want to make several copies of the plan: one for you, one for your chart, one for your doctor or nurse-midwife, and one for your birthing coach or partner. And bringing a few extra copies in your labor bag is a good idea, especially if your doctor ends up not being on call when your baby is born.

Although you may not be able to control everything that happens to you during your baby's birth, you can play a role in the decisions that are made about your body and your baby. A well thought-out birth plan can help you to do that.

Chapter 40

Choosing A Birth Location

There are plenty of decisions to consider during pregnancy. Opting for prenatal testing, selecting a doctor for your baby, and deciding who will be present during your baby's birth are among the more challenging decisions you'll need to make. But where you choose to give birth—whether in a hospital or in a birth center setting—is one of the most important decisions you'll make before delivery.

Hospitals

Many women fear that a typical hospital setting will be a cold and clinical environment, but that's not necessarily always the case. A hospital setting can accommodate a variety of birth experiences.

Traditional hospital births (in which the mother-to-be moves from a labor room to a delivery room and then, after the birth, to a semiprivate room) are still the most common option. In a traditional hospital birth, doctors "manage" the delivery with their patients. In many cases, women in labor are not allowed to eat or drink (possibly due to anesthesia or for other medical reasons), and they may be required to deliver in a certain position. Pain medications are available during

About This Chapter: This information, from "Birthing Centers and Hospital Maternity Services," was provided by KidsHealth, one of the largest resources online for medically reviewed health information written for parents, kids, and teens. For more articles like this one, visit www.KidsHealth.org, or www.TeensHealth.org. © 2005 The Nemours Foundation.

labor and delivery (if the woman chooses); labor may be induced, if necessary; and the fetus is usually electronically monitored throughout the labor. Of course, a birth plan can help a woman communicate her preferences about these issues, and most doctors will be as accommodating as possible.

In response to a push for more "natural" birth events, many hospitals now offer more modern options for low-risk births, often known as family-centered care. These may include private rooms with baths (known as birthing suites) where women can labor, deliver, and recover in one place without having to be moved. Although a doctor and medical staff are still present, the rooms are usually set up to create a nurturing environment, with warm, soothing colors, and amenities that try to simulate a home-like atmosphere that may be very comforting for some new mothers. Rooming in—when the baby stays with the mother most of the time instead of in the infant nursery—may also be available.

In addition, many hospitals offer a variety of childbirth and prenatal education classes to prepare parents for the birth experience, as well as parenting classes after birth.

The number of people allowed to attend the birth varies from hospital to hospital. In more traditional settings, as many as three support people are permitted to be with the mother during a vaginal birth. In a family-centered approach, more family members, friends, and sometimes, even children, may be allowed. During a routine or non-emergency cesarean section, the number of support people is usually limited to one.

If you decide to give birth in a hospital, you will encounter a variety of health professionals.

Obstetrician/gynecologists (OB/GYNs) are doctors with at least four additional years of training after medical school in women's health and reproduction, including both surgical and medical care. They can handle complicated pregnancies and can also perform cesarean sections.

Look for obstetricians who are board-certified, meaning they have passed an examination by the American Board of Obstetrics and Gynecology. Some board-certified obstetricians go on to then receive further training in high-risk pregnancies. These physicians are called maternal-fetal specialists or perinatologists.

If you deliver in a hospital, you may also be able to use a certified nurse-midwife (CNM). CNMs are registered nurses who have a graduate degree in midwifery, meaning they are trained to handle normal, low-risk pregnancies and deliveries. Most CNMs deliver babies in hospitals or birth centers, although some do home births.

In addition to obstetricians and CNMs, registered nurses are typically present during a birth to take care of the mother and baby. If you give birth in a teaching hospital, medical students or residents may also be present during the birth. Some family doctors also offer prenatal care and deliver babies.

While you are in the hospital, if you choose or if it's necessary for you to receive anesthesia, it will be administered by a trained anesthesiologist. A variety of pain control measures, including pain medication and local, epidural, and general anesthesia, are also available in the hospital setting.

Birth Centers

Women who experience delivery in a birth center are usually those who have already given birth without any problems and whose current pregnancies are considered low risk (meaning they are in good health and are the least likely to develop complications). A woman who's giving birth to multiples, who has certain medical conditions such as gestational diabetes or high blood pressure, or whose baby is in the breech position would be considered higher risk and should not deliver in a birth center. Women are carefully screened early in pregnancy and are given prenatal care at the birth center to monitor their health throughout their pregnancy.

Natural childbirth is the focus in a birth center. Since epidural anesthesia is not typically offered, women are free to move around in labor, get in positions that are most comfortable to them, spend time in the Jacuzzi; in other words, deal with the labor in a proactive manner. The baby is monitored frequently in labor typically with a handheld Doppler. Comfort measures such as hydrotherapy, massage, warm and cold compresses, and visualization and relaxation techniques are often used. The woman is free to eat and drink as she chooses.

A variety of health care professionals operate in the birth center setting. A birth center may employ registered nurses, CNMs, and doulas (professionally trained providers of labor support and/or postpartum care). Although a doctor is seldom present and medical interventions are rarely done, birth centers may work with a variety of obstetric and pediatric consultants. The professionals affiliated with a birth center work closely together as a team, with the nurse-midwives present and the OB/GYN consultants being available if a woman develops a complication during pregnancy or labor that puts her into a higher risk category.

Birth centers typically do have medical equipment available, including intravenous lines and fluids, oxygen for the mother and the infant, infant resuscitators, infant warmers, local anesthesia to repair tears and episiotomies (although these are seldom performed), and oxytocin to control postpartum bleeding. A birth center can provide natural pain control and pain control with mild narcotic medications, but if a woman decides she wants an epidural, or if complications develop, she must be taken to the hospital.

Birth centers often provide a homey birth experience for the mother, baby, and extended family. In most cases, birth centers are freestanding buildings, although they may be attached to a hospital. Birth centers may be located in residential areas and generally include amenities such as private rooms with soft lighting, showers, and whirlpool tubs. A kitchen may be available for the family to use.

Look for a birth center that is accredited by the Commission for the Accreditation of Birth Centers (CABC). Some states regulate birth centers, so you may want to find out whether the birth center you choose has all the proper credentials.

Which One Is Right For You?

How do you decide whether a hospital or a birth center is the right choice for you? If you've chosen a particular health care provider, he or she may only practice at a particular hospital or birth center, so you should discuss your decision with him or her. You should also verify your choice with your health insurance carrier to make sure that your prospective hospital or birth center is covered. In many cases, accredited birth centers as well as hospitals, are covered by major insurance companies.

If you have any conditions that would classify your pregnancy as higher risk (such as being older than 35, carrying multiple fetuses, or having gestational diabetes or high blood pressure, to name a few), your health care provider may advise you to have your child in a hospital where you and your baby can receive the required medical treatment, if necessary. In fact, you may be ineligible to deliver in a birth center because of your risk factors.

If you desire interventions such as an epidural or continuous fetal monitoring, a hospital is probably the better choice for you.

For a woman without significant problems in her medical history and whose pregnancy has been classified as low risk, a birth center might be an option. Someone who desires a natural birth with minimal medical intervention or pain control may feel more comfortable in a birth center. Because the number of labor and support people you can choose to be present is less limited, if you want to have your entire family participate in the birthing experience, you might consider a birth center.

Choosing A Hospital Or Birth Center

Once you've decided on either a hospital or a birth center, you may still have to choose which hospital or which birth center. Before you make a choice, you'll have to verify if your health care provider, whether he or she is

♣ It's A Fact!!
Homebirth

Pregnant women with no risk factors for complications during pregnancy, labor, or delivery can consider a homebirth. You should ask your insurance company about their policy on homebirths.

To ensure your safety and that of your baby, you must have a highly trained and experienced midwife along with a fail-safe back-up plan.

Source: Excerpted from "Labor and Birth," National Women's Health Information Center, U.S. Department of Health and Human Services, January 2006.

a doctor or a CNM, will only deliver at certain facilities. In addition, it's a good idea to get a tour of the hospital or birth center so you can determine for yourself if the staff is friendly and the atmosphere is one in which you will feel relaxed.

Before your labor pains start, get answers to the following questions.

Choosing A Hospital: Questions To Ask

- Is the hospital easy to get to?

- How is it equipped to handle emergencies?

- What level nursery is available? (Nurseries are rated I, II, or III—a level III neonatal intensive care unit (NICU) is equipped to handle any neonatal emergency. A lower rating may require transportation to a level III NICU.)

- How many deliveries take place at the hospital each year? (A higher number means the hospital has more experience with various birth scenarios.)

- What is the nurse-to-patient ratio? (A ratio of 1:2 is considered good during low-risk labor; a 1:1 ratio is best in complicated cases or during the pushing stage.)

- What are the hospital's statistics for cesarean sections, episiotomies, and

---

**✔ Quick Tip
Packing For The
Hospital**

Here are some suggestions of items to pack for yourself, your coach, and your baby. It's a good idea to pack several weeks before your due date in case you go into labor early.

For You

- bras (2)

- nightgown (nursing)

- robe and slippers

- socks (several pairs)

- toiletries

- hair dryer

- calling card for phone/ change for pay phone

- going home clothes (in a size that fit during your sixth month of pregnancy)

For Your Baby

- baby clothes

- hat

- receiving blanket

- warm over-clothes (depending on the weather)

- car seat

For Your Labor And Delivery Bag

- tapes of favorite music

- contact lens case and eye-glasses
- breathing sheet and coach's guide
- two or more pillows with bright colored cases
- two colored washcloths
- lip balm
- mouthwash, toothbrush, and toothpaste
- pair of socks
- snacks and beverages for coach
- focal point
- powder and/or lotion for massage
- barrettes and hair wrap
- tennis balls in a sock
- camera and extra film, video recorder
- change for pay phone and vending machines
- magazine, games
- paper and pencil
- list of phone numbers of people to notify of birth

Source: "Packing for the Hospital," © 2006 Northwest Community Healthcare. All rights reserved. Reprinted with permission.

mortality? (Keep in mind, though, that these numbers include high-risk and complicated deliveries.)

- How many labor and support people may be present for the birth?
- What procedures are followed after your baby's birth? Can you breastfeed immediately if desired? Is rooming in available?
- How long is the typical postpartum stay for vaginal deliveries? For cesarean sections?
- Can the baby and the father stay with you in your room around the clock, if you desire?

Choosing A Birth Center: Questions To Ask

- Is the birth center accredited by the Commission for the Accreditation of Birth Centers?
- Is the birth center easy to get to?
- What situations during labor would lead to a transfer to a hospital? How are transfers handled? What emergencies are the transfer facilities able to handle?
- What professionals (such as midwives, doctors, and nurses) are available on staff? On a consulting basis? Are they licensed?
- What childbirth and prenatal education classes are offered?

- What are the center's statistics for hospital transfers, episiotomies, and mortality?

- What procedures are followed after your baby's birth? How long is the typical postpartum stay and how will your baby be examined?

Choosing where to deliver your baby is a complicated decision and one you'll want to decide upon as early in your pregnancy as possible. That way, if complications do arise, you'll be well informed, and you can concentrate on your health and the health of your baby instead of making last-minute decisions.

Chapter 41

Signs Of Labor

What Is Labor?

Labor is the process by which contractions of a pregnant uterus cause birth. During labor, the cervix thins (effaces) and opens (dilation). The baby moves down the birth canal and is born. Delivery of the placenta is the last part of labor.

Every labor is different. How long it lasts and how it progresses differ from woman to woman and from birth to birth. There are, however, general guidelines for labor that a health care provider uses to decide whether it is progressing normally. If it is not progressing normally, you may need medical assistance or a cesarean section.

No one knows exactly what starts the labor process. However, we do know that certain hormones, such as oxytocin and prostaglandin, cause uterine contractions and the thinning of the cervix.

How To Tell When Labor Is Approaching

Some changes take place that may signal the approach of labor. These changes are listed in Table 41.1. Except for the contractions, you may or may not notice some of these signs before labor begins.

About This Chapter: Information in this chapter is from "How to Tell When Labor Begins." Reprinted with permission from the University of Michigan Health System, www.med.umich.edu. Copyright © 2005 Regents of the University of Michigan.

Table 41.1. Signs That You Are Approaching Labor

Sign	What It Is	When It Happens
Feeling as if the baby has dropped lower.	Lightening. Commonly referred to as the "baby dropping." The baby's head has settled deep into your pelvis.	From a few weeks to a few hours before labor begins.
Discharging a thick plug of mucus or having an increase of vaginal discharge (clear, pink, or slightly bloody).	Show. A thick mucus plug has accumulated at the cervix during pregnancy. When the cervix begins to open, the plug is pushed into the vagina.	Several days before labor begins or at the onset of labor.
Discharging a continuous trickle or a gush of watery fluid from your vagina.	Rupture of the membranes. The fluid filled sac that surrounded the baby during pregnancy breaks (your "water breaks").	From several hours before labor begins to any time during labor.
Feeling a regular pattern of cramps or what may feel like a bad backache or menstrual cramps.	Contractions. Your uterus is muscle that tightens and relaxes. The hardness you feel is from your uterus contracting. These contractions may cause pain as the cervix opens and the baby moves through the birth canal.	Usually at the onset of labor.

True Labor Versus False Labor

In the last several weeks of pregnancy, you may notice that your abdomen gets hard and then gets soft again. As you get closer to your delivery date, you may find that this becomes uncomfortable or even painful. These irregular cramps are called Braxton-Hicks contractions, or false labor pains. They may occur more frequently when you are physically active.

False labor can occur just at the time when labor is expected to start. Thus, it is sometimes difficult to tell this from true labor. Don't be upset or embarrassed if you react by thinking labor is beginning. Sometimes the difference can only be determined by a vaginal exam—changes in your cervix signal the onset of true, active labor. Other times, there are ways that might help you to tell the difference between true and false labor.

✔ **Quick Tip**

It's best to be cautious—don't wait too long to call your health care provider if you think you are going into labor.

One good way to tell is to time the contractions. Time how long each cramping period lasts and the length of time in between each contraction. Keep a record for an hour. During true labor the following happens:

- The contractions last about 50–80 seconds.

- They occur at regular intervals.

- They don't go away when you move around.

Call your health care provider when contractions reach the level that you agreed upon earlier as the time to call.

Keep in mind that it can be hard to time labor pains accurately if the contractions are slight.

Chapter 42

Pain Relief During Labor

A concern that most pregnant women have is how they will cope with the pain of labor and childbirth. Because you cannot tell in advance how much pain or discomfort you will have during birth or how you will cope with it, you should think about the possibility that you may need some form of pain relief.

Your preferences will be taken into account in deciding what type of pain relief is best for you, but many other factors, including your well-being and that of your baby, will affect this choice. Keep in mind that often your health care provider will not be able to tell you exactly what kind of pain relief you will receive until you are in labor or are ready to deliver. Many times these choices must be left open and flexible until your health care provider sees how your labor is going. Also, you may not always be able to have medication just when you feel you need it.

Types Of Pain Relief

Having pain, or getting relief for it, should not be thought of as a sign of failure or a reason for guilt. Each person's perception of pain is unique. Each woman's labor will be different, and everyone experiences pain differently. That is why it is important that the decision you make about pain relief be the right one for you.

About This Chapter: Information in this chapter is reprinted with permission from the University of Michigan Health System, www.med.umich.edu. Copyright © 2005 Regents of the University of Michigan.

Behavioral Techniques

Many women take childbirth preparation classes in order to learn what to expect during labor and delivery, as well as breathing methods, relaxation techniques, and other ways of coping with pain and discomfort during childbirth. These classes can be quite valuable, and some women are able to use these techniques to get through childbirth without the need for pain medication. Other women find that using these techniques combined with some medications is helpful in relieving the discomfort of labor and birth. Throughout delivery, your health care provider(s) will be available to you to provide reassurance and suggestions for relief of pain.

Childbirth preparation techniques can help a woman manage pain during labor and birth, but they usually do not completely remove it. If, while using these techniques, you still have a level of pain that you are unwilling or unable to tolerate, pain relief medication is available. It is up to you and your health care provider to weigh the risks and benefits of each method of pain relief.

Pain Relief Medications

Pain-relieving medications fall into two general categories:

- Analgesia is the relief of pain without total loss of sensation. A person receiving an analgesic medication usually remains conscious. While analgesics do not completely stop pain, they do lessen it.

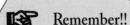 **Remember!!**

Keep in mind that not all types of pain medications are available at all institutions, and not all health care providers are able to give every type.

- Anesthesia refers to the loss of sensation. You will not lose consciousness unless you are given general anesthesia, which is usually reserved for cesarean or emergent delivery.

The decision to use a pain medication and what type to use will depend on several factors. Your health care provider may work with an anesthesiologist, a health care provider who specializes in pain relief, in selecting the best method for you, depending on how your labor or delivery is going and what your state of health is. Of course, the effect of the medication on your baby must also be considered.

Systemic Analgesia

Systemic analgesics provide pain relief over the entire body without causing loss of consciousness. They act on the whole nervous system, rather than on one particular area. Systemic analgesics are often given as an injection into a muscle or vein. Sometimes other drugs are given with systemic analgesics to relieve tension or nausea. While systemic analgesics do not completely get rid of pain, they do lessen its intensity.

Systemic analgesics may cause drowsiness and may make it hard to concentrate. Because these drugs can slow the baby's reflexes and breathing at birth, they are usually avoided just before delivery.

Epidural Block

Epidural block, another form of local anesthesia, affects a much larger area than any of the methods described above. It numbs the lower half of the body to a varying extent, based on the drug and dose used. An epidural block is injected into the lower back, where the nerves that receive sensations from the lower body meet the spinal cord. This kind of anesthesia is helpful for easing the pain of uterine contractions, the pain in the vagina and rectum as the baby descends, and the pain of an episiotomy. While the drug is working, though, you may lose some muscle control in these areas, making it harder to "bear down" during delivery or to move your legs. Epidural blocks are also effective in blocking pain during cesarean birth—delivery of the baby through a surgical incision made in the mother's abdomen and uterus.

An epidural block is injected into a small space around the spinal cord in the lower back. You will be asked to sit or lie on your side with your back curved outward, and to hold this position until the procedure is complete. It may take a while for the drug to take effect. After the needle is inserted, a small tube may be inserted through it, and the needle will then be withdrawn. That way, small doses can be given through the tube at a later time without your having to have another injection. These smaller doses are less likely to cause side effects in the mother and the baby.

Epidural block can have some side effects. It may cause the mother's blood pressure to drop, which in turn may slow the baby's heartbeat. Usually, preventive steps are taken to avoid this problem. Before the mother receives the medication, fluids are given through an intravenous, or IV, line (a thin tube attached to a needle in a vein) in her arm, and she is positioned on her side to help circulation.

With epidural analgesia, it may be harder for the mother to bear down and help the baby move through the birth canal. It may be necessary for the baby to be delivered with forceps or vacuum extraction, special instruments that are placed around or attached to the baby's head to help guide it out of the birth canal.

If the covering of the spinal cord is punctured when the drug is given, the drug may enter the spinal fluid or a vein. The patient may then get a severe headache, which can last for a day or more. In rare cases, the muscles in the patient's chest may be temporarily affected, causing breathing problems. If the drug enters a vein, it could cause dizziness or, rarely, seizures. Special precautions are taken to avoid these problems.

Epidural block is not for every patient. If a woman is bleeding heavily or if the baby has an abnormal heartbeat, epidural blocks may not be used.

Spinal Block

A spinal block, like an epidural block, is given as an injection in the lower back. However, a spinal block has to be injected into the spinal fluid, so the needle is inserted a little deeper (though it does not touch the spinal cord itself). Because the effects of the drug do not last long, and because a spinal block is usually given only once, this form of anesthesia is best suited for pain relief during delivery (not labor), particularly if forceps or vacuum extraction is needed. It is the pain relief method most often used for cesarean birth.

A spinal block numbs the lower half of the body. It provides good relief from pain, starts working quickly, and is effective in small doses.

Spinal block can sometimes cause some of the same side effects as epidural block such as headaches or a drop in the mother's blood pressure and the baby's heartbeat.

Local Anesthesia

Just as a dentist will inject a drug into your gums to numb your teeth, your health care provider can inject a local anesthetic into the vagina or the area surrounding it to ease pain during delivery. Local anesthetics usually affect a small area, and so are especially useful when the health care provider has to make an episiotomy, a small cut, or incision, made in the perineum (the area between the vagina and the rectum) before the baby passes through. Local anesthetics are also helpful when this incision, or any tears that might have occurred during birth, are repaired.

One advantage of local anesthesia is that it rarely affects the baby. After the anesthetic wears off, there are usually no lingering effects. The main drawback of these drugs is that they do not relieve the pain of contractions during labor.

General Anesthesia

General anesthetics are medications that make you lose consciousness. When general anesthesia is used during childbirth, the mother will not be awake or feel any pain during delivery. It is not used to relieve the pain of labor. General anesthesia is rarely used for routine vaginal deliveries. It is often used for cesarean delivery or other urgent situations.

These drugs are given in one of two ways: through a face mask or injected through an IV line. Once the drug is given, it works very quickly, and is usually given just before delivery.

When general anesthetics are used during childbirth, the patient's stomach may not be empty. While she is under anesthesia she may vomit and breathe in food and stomach acid, which can harm her lungs and cause pneumonia. There are some precautions that will help avoid this complication. Your health care provider may tell you not to eat anything once labor begins. If general anesthesia is likely to be used, you may be given an antacid before delivery. After you are asleep, a tube will probably be placed in your throat to help you breathe.

General anesthesia is not a good choice for some women. Serious side effects, though rare, can occur. Be sure to tell your health care provider if you or anyone in your family has ever had a drug reaction or a problem with any form of anesthesia.

After general anesthesia wears off, you will feel woozy and tired for several hours after waking up. You may also feel sick to your stomach; this feeling usually fades within a day. Also, your throat may be sore from the tube that was inserted to provide oxygen.

Recovery From Pain Medications

What you experience as you recover from pain medications will depend on the type that was used. In any case, once it wears off, you may feel some pain around the vagina, perineum, lower abdomen, or back, depending on how much the muscles and tissues were strained during delivery. If you are in pain, ask your health care provider if you can get some medication.

☞ Remember!!

Many women worry that anesthesia given during labor or childbirth will somehow make the experience less "natural." The fact is, no two labors or deliveries are the same, and no two people have exactly the same ability to tolerate pain. Some women require little or no pain medication, while many others find that pain relief gives them a better sense of control over their labor and delivery.

Be prepared to be flexible. Some of the techniques described here may appeal to you more than others, but your health and the health of your baby must be considered when it comes time to decide if a pain medication is needed and, if so, which one will be best.

Chapter 43

Vaginal Birth

Vaginal birth is the term used to describe any delivery of the baby through the vagina (versus a C-section delivery). The baby typically comes through head first. If the baby is not head first, (e.g., breech) it may need to be delivered by C-section.

Your body makes some amazing changes in the days and hours leading up to your baby's birth.

A day or two before labor begins, the mucus plug that sealed off your uterus detaches from the cervix and passes through your vagina. This discharge is sometimes called "bloody show" because it is tinged with blood.

Before labor begins or in the early stages of labor, your amniotic sac may rupture and you may feel fluid trickle or gush out of your vagina. If your "bag of waters" doesn't break on its own, your doctor may rupture it manually.

Explore your pain relief options before you go into labor. Some women aim for a drug-free delivery and rely on various breathing techniques, massage, visualization, hypnosis, and other strategies to ease the pain of labor. Others prefer pain medication or regional anesthesia (such as an epidural, which numbs the lower half of your body).

✎ What's It Mean?

Amniotic Fluid: Clear, slightly yellowish liquid that surrounds the unborn baby (fetus) during pregnancy. It is contained in the amniotic sac.

Amniotic Sac: During pregnancy, the amniotic sac is formed within the uterus and encloses the fetus. This sac bursts normally during the birthing process, releasing the amniotic fluid. A popular term for the amniotic sac with the amniotic fluid is the bag of waters.

Cervix: The lower, narrow part of the uterus (womb). The cervix forms a canal that opens into the vagina, which leads to the outside of the body.

Epidural: During labor a woman may be offered an epidural, where a needle is inserted into the epidural space at the end of the spine, to numb the lower body and reduce pain. This allows a woman to have more energy and strength for the end stage of labor, when it is time to push the baby out of the birth canal.

Placenta: During pregnancy, a temporary organ joining the mother and fetus. The placenta transfers oxygen and nutrients from the mother to the fetus, and permits the release of carbon dioxide and waste products from the fetus. The placenta is expelled during the birth process with the fetal membranes.

Umbilical Cord: Connected to the placenta and provides the transfer of nutrients and waste between the woman and the fetus.

Uterus: A woman's womb, or the hollow, pear-shaped organ located in a woman's lower abdomen between the bladder and the rectum.

Source: "NWHIC Web Site Glossary," National Women's Health Information Center, U.S. Department of Health and Human Services, cited November 2006.

Contractions happen when your uterine muscles involuntarily tighten and relax. When true labor begins, you feel contractions at regular intervals. As labor progresses, these contractions get longer, stronger, and closer together. During active labor, you may feel intense pain or pressure in your back or abdomen during each contraction. You may also feel the urge to push or bear down, though your doctor will ask you to wait until your cervix is completely dilated.

Contractions help your cervix dilate, or open, so your baby can pass through the birth canal. You are fully dilated when your cervical opening measures ten centimeters. As the cervix opens, it also thins (effaces) in preparation for delivery.

When your cervix is fully dilated, your doctor gives you the okay to push. Propelled by your effort and the force of your contractions, the baby makes his way through the birth canal. The fontanels—soft spots—on his head allow it to mold to the shape of this narrow passage. Your baby's head "crowns" when the widest part of it is at the vaginal opening.

As soon as your baby's head emerges, the doctor suctions amniotic fluid, blood, and mucus from his nose and mouth. More contractions and pushing help deliver the baby's shoulders and body.

Unless your partner has requested the honor, the doctor clamps and cuts the umbilical cord and examines your newborn.

It is not over yet. After your baby is born, more contractions help you deliver the placenta, or "afterbirth."

Chapter 44

Cesarean Delivery

Having A Cesarean Delivery

Many patients wonder whether they'll need a cesarean. Sometimes your doctor knows the answer before labor even begins—if you have placenta previa, for example, or if the baby is in a transverse lie (that is, the baby is lying sideways within the uterus rather than head-down).

Because a cesarean is a surgical procedure, it's always performed by a doctor. All nurse-midwives and many family practice doctors work with an obstetrician trained to perform cesarean deliveries in case any of their patients need one. Some family practice physicians have had the special training needed to perform cesarean deliveries.

A doctor performs a cesarean delivery in an operating room under sterile conditions. A nurse puts in an intravenous line in the patient's arm and a catheter in the bladder. After a nurse or nurse's assistant scrubs the patient's abdomen with antiseptic solution, a nurse places sterile sheets over the patient's belly. One of the sheets is elevated to create a screen so that the expectant parents don't have to watch the procedure. (Although childbirth is usually an experience shared by both parents, a cesarean delivery is still a surgical operation. Most doctors feel

About This Chapter: Information in this chapter is from *Pregnancy For Dummies, 2nd Edition*, by Joanne Stone, M.D., Keith Eddleman, M.D., Mary Duenwald. Copyright © 2004 by Wiley Publishing Inc. Reprinted with permission of John Wiley and Sons, Inc.

that the procedure isn't something that expectant parents should watch, because it involves scalpels, bleeding, and exposure of internal body tissue that's normally not seen, which is disturbing to many people.)

Many hospitals allow the coach or partner to stay in the operating room during a cesarean delivery, but this decision depends on the nature of the delivery and on hospital policy. If the cesarean is an emergency, the doctors and nurses are moving quickly to ensure the safety of both the mother and the baby, which may make it necessary for the partner or coach to wait elsewhere.

The exact place on the woman's abdomen where the incision is made depends on the reason she's having the cesarean. Most often, it is low, just above the pubic bone, in a transverse direction (perpendicular to the torso). This cut is known as a Pfannenstiel incision or, more commonly, a bikini cut. Less often, the incision is vertical, along the midline of the abdomen.

After the doctor makes the skin incision, he or she separates the abdominal muscles and opens the inner lining of the abdominal cavity, also called the peritoneal cavity, to expose the uterus. He or she then makes an incision in the uterus itself, through which the infant and placenta are delivered. The incision in the uterus can also be either transverse (most common) or vertical (sometimes called a classical incision) depending again on the reason for the cesarean and previous abdominal surgery. After delivery, the uterus and abdominal wall are closed with sutures, layer by layer. A cesarean delivery takes 30 to 90 minutes to perform.

Understanding Anesthesia

The most common forms of anesthesia used for cesarean deliveries are epidural and spinal. Both kinds of anesthesia numb you from mid-chest to toes but also allow you to remain awake so that you can experience your child's birth. You may feel some tugging and pulling during the operation, but you don't feel pain. Sometimes the anesthesiologist injects a slow-release pain medication into the epidural or spinal catheter before removing it in order to prevent or greatly minimize pain after the operation.

If the baby has to be delivered in an emergency and there's no time to place an epidural or spinal, general anesthesia may be needed. In that case, you're asleep during the cesarean and totally unaware of the procedure.

Looking At Reasons For Cesarean Delivery

The reasons your doctor may perform a cesarean delivery are many, but all are about delivering the infant in the safest, healthiest way possible while also maintaining the mother's well-being. A cesarean delivery can be either planned ahead of labor (elective), unplanned during labor (when the doctor determines that delivering the baby vaginally isn't safe), or done as an emergency (if the mother's or the baby's health is in immediate jeopardy).

If your practitioner feels that you need a cesarean delivery, he or she will discuss with you why it is needed. If your cesarean is elective or it's done because your labor isn't progressing normally, you and your partner have time to ask questions. In cases in which the baby is in a breech position, you and your practitioner may consider together the pros and cons of having either an elective cesarean delivery or a vaginal breech delivery. Both carry some risks, and often your practitioner asks you which risks are most acceptable to you. If the decision to perform a cesarean is due to a last-minute emergency, the discussion between you and your doctor may happen quickly, while you're being wheeled to the operating room.

If things seem hurried or rushed when you're on your way to the operating room for an emergency cesarean, don't panic. Doctors and nurses are trained to handle these kinds of emergencies.

♣ It's A Fact!!
General anesthesia may be needed in some cases because of complications in pregnancy that make it unwise to place epidurals or spinals.

Your practitioner may suggest that you have a cesarean delivery for one of many different reasons. This list describes the most common ones:

- The baby is in an abnormal position (breech or transverse).

- Placenta previa.

- You've had extensive prior surgery on the uterus, including previous cesarean deliveries or removal of uterine fibroids.

- Delivery of triplets or more.

Reasons for unplanned but non-emergency cesarean delivery include the following:

- The baby is too large in relation to the woman's pelvis to be delivered safely through the vagina—a condition known as cephalopelvic disproportion (CPD)—or the position of the baby's head makes vaginal delivery unlikely.

- Signs indicate that the baby isn't tolerating labor.

- Maternal medical conditions preclude safe vaginal delivery, such as severe cardiac disease.

- Normal labor comes to a standstill.

Reasons for emergency cesarean deliveries are as follows:

- Bleeding is excessive.

- The baby's umbilical cord pushes through the cervix when the membranes rupture.

- Prolonged slowing of the baby's heart rate.

Other than the fact that the baby and placenta are delivered through an incision in the uterus rather than through the vagina, a cesarean delivery for the baby is of little difference. Babies delivered by a cesarean before labor usually don't have the cone heads, but they may if you're in labor for a long time before having a cesarean.

Women who have labored for a long time only to find that they need a cesarean delivery are sometimes, understandably, disappointed. This reaction is natural. If it happens to you, keep in mind that what is ultimately most important is your safety and your baby's safety. Having a cesarean delivery doesn't mean that you are, in any way, a failure or that you didn't try hard enough. Practitioners stick to basic guidelines when monitoring progress through labor, and those guidelines are all about giving you and your baby the best chance for a normal, healthy outcome.

All surgical procedures involve risks, and cesarean delivery is no exception. Fortunately, these problems aren't common. The main risks of cesarean delivery are the following:

- Excessive bleeding, rarely to the point of needing a blood transfusion

- Development of an infection in the uterus, bladder, or skin incision

- Injury to the bladder, bowel, or adjacent organs

- Development of blood clots in the legs or pelvis after the operation

Recovering From A Cesarean Delivery

The hospital stay after a cesarean delivery is generally a few days longer than after a vaginal delivery—usually three to four days in total. If you have a cesarean delivery, you're put on a stretcher immediately afterward and transported to the recovery room. You may be able to hold your baby in your arms during the trip.

Going To The Recovery Room

When you're in the recovery room, your nurse and anesthesiologist monitor your vital signs. The nurse periodically checks your abdomen to make sure that the uterus is firm and that the dressing over the incision is dry. Your nurse also checks for signs of excessive bleeding from the uterus. More than likely, you have a catheter in your bladder, and it stays in place for the first night so that you don't have to worry about getting up to go to the bathroom. You also have an intravenous (IV) line in place to receive fluids and any medications your doctor prescribes. If you had an epidural or spinal anesthetic, your legs may still seem a little numb or heavy. This feeling wears off in a few hours. If you had general anesthesia (that is, if you were "put to sleep"), you may feel a little groggy when you get to the recovery room. Just as with a vaginal delivery, you may experience some shaking. If you're up to it and if you want to, you can breastfeed your baby while you're in the recovery room.

Most likely, you receive pain medication in the operating room, and you don't need any more while you're in the recovery room. In some hospitals, if you have an epidural or spinal, your anesthesiologist injects a long-lasting medication into the catheter that keeps you almost pain-free for about 24 hours. If, however, your pain medication doesn't seem to be working, by all means let your nurse know.

Taking It One Step At A Time

When your nurse and anesthesiologist are confident that your vital signs are stable and that you're recovering normally from the anesthesia, you're discharged from the recovery room—generally about one to three hours after delivery. You're transported on a stretcher to a hospital room, where you spend the rest of your recovery time.

The Day Of Delivery: On the day of your cesarean, you should plan on just staying in bed. Thanks to your catheter, you don't need to worry about getting up to go to the bathroom. If you had your surgery early in the morning, you may feel like getting up later in the evening, even if only to sit in a chair. Just be sure to check with your nurse first to see whether getting up is okay. When you get up the first time, make sure that someone is there to help you.

Although some doctors still prefer that patients not have any food immediately after a cesarean, many doctors now allow women to eat and drink shortly after the surgery. Often, the patient is the best judge of what she should and shouldn't do. If you feel queasy and nauseous, you're better off not eating. But if you feel hungry, drinking liquids and having small amounts of solid food is probably fine.

Like women who have had a vaginal delivery, expect some vaginal bleeding (lochia) after a cesarean. The bleeding may be quite heavy during the first few days after your surgery.

The Day After: The first day after your surgery, your doctor is likely to encourage you to get out of bed and start to walk around. The first couple of times you get up to walk may be pretty uncomfortable—you may feel pain around the incision in your abdomen—so you may want to ask for a so-called top up dose of pain medication 20 minutes or so before getting up.

Make sure someone is with you the first few times you get up to make sure that you don't fall.

Depending on your fluid needs, your doctor may also discontinue your IV line. Most of the time, you're able to drink liquids on the first day, and many doctors also let you eat solid food.

Most likely, you have a bandage over your abdominal incision. Sometimes this bandage comes off on day one, but sometimes doctors prefer to leave it on longer.

Many women ask about "rooming in"—that is, having the baby stay in the room with them—after a cesarean delivery, especially after they've had a day or so to recover a bit from the procedure. Having the baby in the room with you is certainly fine if you feel up to it. But by no means feel that you have to. Keep in mind that you just had abdominal surgery, and you may not be physically able to attend to every single one of your baby's needs during the first few days afterward. The hospital nurses are there to help, so during this time devote as much energy as possible to your own recovery. You'll be that much better able to care for your baby after you get home.

♣ It's A Fact!!

Most women who have a cesarean delivery and have staples in their skin worry that removing the staples will hurt. But don't worry. Staple removal is a quick and painless procedure.

Chapter 45

Breech Birth

Usually a few weeks before birth, most babies will move into delivery position with their head moving near the birth canal. If this does not happen, the baby's buttocks and/or feet will be in place to be delivered first. This is called a breech presentation. Breech births occur in about 1 of 25 full-term births.

What are the different types of breech presentations?

- **Frank Breech:** The fetus's buttocks are aimed toward the birth canal and the legs stick straight up in front of the body. The feet are near the head.

- **Complete Breech:** The buttocks are down, with the legs folded at the knees and the feet near the buttocks.

- **Footling Breech:** One or both of the fetus's feet are pointing down and will come out first.

What causes a breech presentation?

The causes of breech presentations are not fully known. However, a breech birth is more common in the following situations:

- in subsequent pregnancies

- in pregnancies of multiples

About This Chapter: Information in this chapter is from "Breech Births," reprinted with permission from the American Pregnancy Association, http://www.americanpregnancy.org, © 2006. All rights reserved.

- when there is a history of premature delivery

- when the uterus has too much or too little amniotic fluid

- in an abnormal shaped uterus or a uterus with abnormal growths such as fibroids

- for women with placenta previa

How is a breech presentation diagnosed?

A few weeks prior to the due date, the health care provider may place his/her hands on the mother's lower abdomen to locate the baby's head, back, and buttocks. If they think the baby is in a breech position, an ultrasound may be used to confirm. Special x-rays can also determine the baby's position and measure the pelvis to determine if a vaginal delivery of a breech baby may be attempted.

Can a breech presentation mean something is wrong?

Most breech babies are born healthy. However, they do have a higher risk for certain problems than babies born headfirst. Birth defects are slightly more common in breech babies. A birth defect may be the reason they have not moved into the right position before birth.

Can a breech presentation be changed?

The best time to try to turn a breech baby is between 32–37 weeks of pregnancy. There are many different types of methods to use and all have different levels of success. Talk with your health care provider on which options they feel would be best for you to try.

Medical Techniques

External Version: External version is a non-surgical method in which a doctor can help move the baby within the uterus. A medication to help relax the uterus might be given as well as an ultrasound exam to better check the position of the baby, the location of the placenta, and the amount of amniotic fluid in the uterus. Gentle pushing on the lower abdomen can turn the baby into the head-down position. Throughout the external version, the baby's heartbeat will be checked closely so that if any problems should occur, the doctor will stop turning immediately. Most attempts at external version are successful; however, as the due date gets closer, this procedure is more difficult.

Chiropractic Care: The late Larry Webster, D.C., of the International Chiropractic Pediatric Association, developed a technique which enabled chiropractors to release stress on the pregnant woman's pelvis and cause relaxation to the uterus and surrounding ligaments. The relaxed uterus would make it easier for a breech baby to turn naturally. The technique is known as the Webster Breech Technique.

✔ **Quick Tip**

There are homeopathic remedies that women have found to be successful in breech situations. Contact your local holistic practitioner about the use of moxibustion or pulsatilla in turning breech babies naturally.

The *Journal of Manipulative and Physiological Therapeutics* reported in the July/August 2002 issue that 82% of doctors using the Webster Technique reported success. Further, the results from the study suggest that it may be beneficial to perform the Webster Technique in the 8th month of pregnancy.

Natural Techniques

The following two techniques often suggested by physical therapist, Penny Simkin, are things you can try at home for free, with no risks involved.

The Breech Tilt: Raise hips 12 inches or 30 centimeters off the floor using large, solid pillows three times daily for 10–15 minutes each time. This is best done on an empty stomach and at a time when your baby is active. Concentrate on your baby and not tensing your body, especially in the abdomen area.

Using Music: We know that babies can hear sounds outside the womb, so many women have used music or taped recordings of their voice to try to get their baby to move towards the "noise." Headphones placed on the lower part of your abdomen, playing either music or your voice, has encouraged babies to move towards the sounds and out of the breech position.

Vaginal delivery versus cesarean for breech birth?

Most doctors do not believe a vaginal delivery is possible for a breech birth, although some will wait to make that decision until a woman is in labor. However, the following are often necessary factors in order for a vaginal birth to be attempted, if the care provider is willing:

- The baby is full-term and in the frank breech presentation.
- The baby does not show signs of distress as its heart rate is closely monitored.
- The process of labor is smooth and steady; the cervix is widening and the baby is moving down.
- The doctor estimates that the baby is not too big or the mother's pelvis too narrow for the baby to pass safely through the birth canal.
- Anesthesia is available, and a cesarean delivery can be performed on short notice.

What are the risks and complications of a vaginal delivery?

In a breech birth, the baby's head is the last part to emerge, and it may be harder to ease it through the birth canal. Sometimes forceps are used to guide the baby's head out. Another potential problem is cord prolapse in which the umbilical cord can get squeezed as the baby moves toward the birth canal, slowing the baby's supply of oxygen and blood.

If a vaginal delivery is attempted, electronic fetal monitoring will be used to monitor the baby's heartbeat throughout labor. A cesarean delivery may be considered if there are any signs that the baby may be in distress.

When is a cesarean delivery used with a breech presentation?

Most physicians recommend a cesarean delivery for all babies that are in a breech position, especially those that are premature. Premature babies are small and fragile, and because the head is relatively larger, their bodies do not stretch the cervix as wide as full-term babies do during birth. This means that there may be less room for the head to emerge.

Part Six

Introducing Your Newborn

Chapter 46

The First Few Hours Of Life: Medical Care For Your Newborn

Right after birth, babies need many important tests and procedures to ensure their health. Some of these are even required by law; but as long as the baby is healthy, everything but the Apgar test can wait for at least an hour. Delaying further medical care will preserve the precious few moments of life for you and the baby.

A baby who has not been poked and prodded may be more willing to nurse and cuddle; so before delivery, talk to your doctor or midwife about delaying shots, medicine, and tests.

The following tests and procedures are recommended or required in most hospitals in the United States:

- Apgar evaluation

- eye care

- vitamin K shot

- newborn metabolic screening

- hearing test

About This Chapter: Information in this chapter is from "Right after Birth," National Women's Health Information Center, U.S. Department of Health and Human Services, January 2006.

- hepatitis B vaccine

- complete checkup

Apgar Evaluation

The Apgar test is a quick way for doctors to figure out if the baby is healthy or needs extra medical care. Apgar tests are usually done twice, one minute after birth and again five minutes after birth. Doctors and nurses measure five signs of the baby's condition. They are the following:

- heart rate

- breathing

- activity and muscle tone

- reflexes

- skin color

Apgar scores range from 0 to 10. A baby who scores 7 or more is considered very healthy; but a lower score does not always mean there is something wrong. Perfectly healthy babies often have low Apgar scores in the first minute of life.

In more than 98% of cases, the Apgar score reaches 7 after five minutes of life. When it does not, the baby needs medical care and close monitoring.

Eye Care

The Centers for Disease Control and Prevention (CDC) recommend that all newborns receive eye drops or ointment to prevent infections they can get during delivery. Sexually transmitted diseases (STDs) including gonorrhea and chlamydia are a main cause of newborn eye infections. These infections can cause blindness when left untreated.

Silver nitrate, erythromycin, and tetracycline are the three medicines used in newborns' eyes. These medicines can sting and/or blur the baby's vision, so you may want to postpone this treatment for a little while.

Some parents question whether this treatment is really necessary. Many women at low risk for STDs do not want their newborns to receive eye medicine, but there is no evidence to suggest that this medicine harms the baby.

It is important to note that even pregnant women who test negative for STDs may get an infection by the time of delivery. Plus, most women with gonorrhea and/or chlamydia do not know it because they have no symptoms.

Vitamin K Shot

The American Academy of Pediatrics recommends that all newborns receive a shot of vitamin K in the upper leg. Newborns usually have low levels of vitamin K in their bodies. This vitamin is needed for the blood to clot. Low levels of vitamin K can cause a rare, but serious, bleeding problem. Research shows that vitamin K shots prevent dangerous bleeding in newborns.

Newborns probably feel pain when the shot is given; but afterwards, babies do not seem to have any discomfort. Since it may be uncomfortable for the baby, you may want to postpone this shot for a little while.

Newborn Metabolic Screening

Doctors or nurses prick your baby's heel to take a tiny sample of blood. They use this blood to test for many diseases.

All 50 states require testing for at least two disorders, phenylketonuria and congenital hypothyroidism; but many states test for up to 30 different diseases. All of these problems are impossible to spot without a blood test; and if left untreated, they can cause mental retardation and even death.

Hearing Test

Many hospitals offer newborn hearing tests. Tiny earphones or microphones are used to see how the baby reacts to sounds. Newborn hearing tests can spot hearing problems early. This can help cut the risk of serious language and speech problems.

♣ **It's A Fact!!**
The March of Dimes recommends that all newborns be tested for at least 29 diseases.

Hepatitis B Vaccine

Most hospitals now suggest that newborns get a vaccine to protect against the hepatitis B virus

(HBV). HBV can cause a lifelong infection, serious liver damage, and even death.

The hepatitis B vaccine is a series of three different shots. The American Academy of Pediatrics and the Centers for Disease Control and Prevention (CDC) recommend that all newborns get the first shot soon after birth or before leaving the hospital. If the mother does not have hepatitis B, the first shot can wait for two months. The second and last shot should be given before 18 months of age.

Complete Checkup

Soon after delivery, most doctors or nurses also do the following:

- Measure the newborn's weight, length, and head.

- Take the baby's temperature.

- Measure his breathing and heart rates.

- Give the baby a bath and clean the umbilical cord stump.

Chapter 47

Newborn Screening Tests

Newborn screening is the practice of testing every newborn for certain harmful or potentially fatal disorders that aren't otherwise apparent at birth. Many of these are metabolic disorders, often called "inborn errors of metabolism," which interfere with the body's use of nutrients to maintain healthy tissues and produce energy. Other disorders that may be detected through screening include problems with hormones or the blood.

With a simple blood test, doctors can often tell whether newborns have certain conditions that could eventually cause problems. Even though these conditions are considered rare and most babies are given a clean bill of health, early diagnosis and proper treatment can make the difference between life-long impairment and healthy development.

Newborn Screening: Past, Present, And Future

In the early 1960s, scientist Robert Guthrie, PhD, developed a blood test that could determine whether newborn babies had a metabolic disorder known as phenylketonuria (PKU). People with PKU lack an enzyme needed to process the amino acid phenylalanine. This amino acid is necessary for normal

About This Chapter: This information was provided by KidsHealth, one of the largest resources online for medically reviewed health information written for parents, kids, and teens. For more articles like this one, visit www.KidsHealth.org, or www.TeensHealth.org. © 2006 The Nemours Foundation.

growth in infants and children and for normal protein use throughout life. However, if too much of it builds up, it damages the brain tissue and can eventually cause mental retardation.

When babies with PKU are put on a special diet right away, they can often avoid the mental retardation that children with PKU experienced in the past. By following certain dietary restrictions, these children can lead normal lives.

> ♣ **It's A Fact!!**
> In general, metabolic, and other inherited disorders can hinder an infant's normal physical and mental development in a variety of ways, and parents can pass along the gene for a certain disorder without even knowing that they're carriers.

Since the development of the PKU test, researchers have developed additional blood tests that can screen newborns for other disorders that, unless detected and treated early, can cause physical problems, mental retardation, and in some cases, death.

Most states, the District of Columbia, Puerto Rico, and the U.S. Virgin Islands now have their own mandatory newborn screening programs (in some states, such as Wyoming and Maryland, the screening is not mandatory). Because the federal government has set no national standard, screening requirements vary from state to state, as determined by individual state public health departments.

Consequently, the comprehensiveness of these programs varies, with states routinely screening for anywhere from four to 30 disorders. The average state program tests from four to 10 disorders.

State requirements tend to change periodically as well. In fact, the pace of change is speeding up, thanks to the development of a new screening technique known as tandem mass spectrometry (often abbreviated as MS/MS). This technology can detect the blood components that are elevated in certain disorders and is capable of screening for more than 20 inherited metabolic disorders with a single test.

About half of the states are offering expanded screening with tandem mass spectrometry on every baby. However, there's some controversy over whether the new technology has been tested adequately. Also, some experts want more evidence that early detection of every disease tested for will actually offer babies some long-term benefit. Equally important, parents may not want to know ahead of time that their child will develop a serious condition when there are no medical treatments or dietary changes that can improve the outcome, and some questions about who will pay (states, insurance companies, or parents) for the newer technology have yet to be resolved.

The American Academy of Pediatrics (AAP) and the federal government's Health Resources and Services Administration convened a task force of experts to grapple with these issues and recommend next steps. Their report identified some flaws and inconsistencies in the current state-driven screening system and proposed the following:

- All state screening programs should reflect current technology.

- All states should test for the same disorders.

- Parents should be informed about screening procedures and have the right to refuse screening, as well as the right to keep the results private and confidential.

- Parents should be informed about the benefits and risks associated with newborn screening.

All of this can be a little confusing (and anxiety-provoking) for a new parent. The inconsistencies among state requirements mean that there's no clear consensus on what's really necessary. On the one hand, it's important to keep in mind that the disorders being screened for are rare. On the other hand, no parent wants to take any unnecessary chances with the quality of his or her child's life no matter how small the risk.

How Do States And Hospitals Determine Which Tests They Offer?

Traditionally, state decisions about what to screen for have been based on weighing the costs against the benefits. "Cost" considerations include the following:

- the risk of false positive results (and the unnecessary anxiety they cause)

- the availability of treatments proven to help the condition

- financial costs

And states often face conflicting priorities when determining their budgets. For instance, a state may face a choice between expanding newborn screening and ensuring that all expectant mothers get sufficient prenatal care. Of course, this offers little comfort to parents whose children have a disorder that could have been found through a screening test but wasn't.

So what can you do? Your best strategy is to stay informed. Discuss this issue with both your obstetrician or health care provider and your future baby's doctor before you give birth. Know what tests are routinely done in your state and in the hospital where you'll deliver (some hospitals go beyond what's required by state law).

If your state isn't offering screening for the expanded panel of disorders, you may want to ask your doctors about supplemental screening. Keep in mind, though, that you'll probably have to pay for the additional tests out of your own pocket.

What Disorders Will Be Screened For In My Newborn?

Newborn screening varies by state and is subject to change, especially given advancements in technology. However, the disorders listed here are the ones typically included in newborn screening programs and are listed in order from the most common (all states screen for the first two) to least common (ranging from three-fourths or one-half of states to just a few). Incidence figures included in this list are according to a 1996 AAP policy statement.

✔ Quick Tip

If you're the parent of an infant and are concerned about whether your child was screened for certain conditions, ask your child's doctor for information about which tests were performed and whether further tests are recommended.

- **PKU:** When this disorder is detected early, feeding an infant a special formula low in phenylalanine can prevent mental retardation. A low-phenylalanine diet will need to be followed throughout childhood and adolescence and perhaps into adult life. This diet cuts out all high-protein foods, so people with PKU often need to take a special artificial formula as a nutritional substitute. Incidence: 1 in 10,000 to 25,000.

- **Congenital Hypothyroidism:** This is the disorder most commonly identified by routine screening. Affected babies don't have enough thyroid hormone and so develop retarded growth and brain development. (The thyroid, a gland at the front of the neck, releases chemical substances that control metabolism and growth.) If the disorder is detected early, a baby can be treated with oral doses of thyroid hormone to permit normal development. Incidence: 1 in 4,000.

- **Galactosemia:** Babies with galactosemia lack the enzyme that converts galactose (one of two sugars found in lactose) into glucose, a sugar the body is able to use. As a result, milk (including breast milk) and other dairy products must be eliminated from the diet. Otherwise, galactose can build up in the system and damage the body's cells and organs, leading to blindness, severe mental retardation, growth deficiency, and even death. Incidence: 1 in 60,000 to 80,000. There are several less severe forms of galactosemia that may be detected by newborn screening. These may not require any intervention.

- **Sickle Cell Disease:** Sickle cell disease is an inherited blood disease in which red blood cells stretch into abnormal "sickle" shapes and can cause episodes of pain, damage to vital organs such as the lungs and kidneys, and even death. Young children with sickle cell disease are especially prone to certain dangerous bacterial infections, such as pneumonia (inflammation of the lungs) and meningitis (inflammation of the brain and spinal cord). Studies suggest that newborn screening can alert doctors to begin antibiotic treatment before infections occur and to monitor symptoms of possible worsening more closely. The screening test can also detect other disorders affecting hemoglobin (the oxygen-carrying substance in the blood). Incidence: about 1 in every 500 African-American births and 1 in every 1,000 to 1,400 Hispanic American births; also occurs with some frequency among people of Hispanic, Mediterranean, Middle Eastern, and South Asian descent.

- **Biotinidase Deficiency:** Babies with this condition don't have enough biotinidase, an enzyme that recycles biotin (one of the B vitamins) in the body. The deficiency may cause seizures, poor muscle control, immune system impairment, hearing loss, mental retardation, coma, and even death. If the deficiency is detected in time, however, problems can be prevented by giving the baby extra biotin. Incidence: 1 in 72,000 to 126,000.

- **Congenital Adrenal Hyperplasia:** This is actually a group of disorders involving a deficiency of certain hormones produced by the adrenal gland. It can affect the development of the genitals and may cause death due to loss of salt from the kidneys. Lifelong treatment through supplementation of the missing hormones manages the condition. Incidence: 1 in 12,000.

- **Maple Syrup Urine Disease (MSUD):** Babies with MSUD are missing an enzyme needed to process three amino acids that are essential for the body's normal growth. When these are not processed properly, they can build up in the body, causing urine to smell like maple syrup or sweet, burnt sugar. These babies usually have little appetite and are extremely irritable. If not detected and treated early, MSUD can cause mental retardation, physical disability, and even death. A carefully controlled diet that cuts out certain high-protein foods containing those amino acids can prevent these outcomes. Like people with PKU, those with MSUD are often given a formula that supplies the necessary nutrients missed in the special diet they must follow. Incidence: 1 in 250,000.

- **Homocystinuria:** This metabolic disorder results from a deficiency of one of several enzymes for normal development. If untreated, it can lead to dislocated lenses of the eyes, mental retardation, skeletal abnormalities, and abnormal blood clotting. However, a special diet combined with dietary supplements may help prevent most of these problems. Incidence: 1 in 50,000 to 150,000.

- **Tyrosinemia:** Babies with this disorder have trouble processing the amino acid tyrosine. If it accumulates in the body, it can cause mild retardation, language skill difficulties, liver problems, and even death from liver failure.

A special diet and sometimes a liver transplant are needed to treat the condition. Early diagnosis and treatment seem to offset long-term problems, although more information is needed. Incidence: not yet determined. Some babies have a mild self-limited form of tyrosinemia.

- **Cystic Fibrosis:** Cystic fibrosis is an inherited disorder expressed in the various organs that causes cells to release a thick mucus, which can lead to chronic respiratory disease, problems with digestion, and poor growth. There is no known cure—treatment involves trying to prevent the serious lung infections associated with it and providing adequate nutrition. Some infections may be prevented with antibiotics. Detecting the disease early may help doctors reduce the lung and nutritional problems associated with cystic fibrosis, but the real impact of newborn screening is yet to be determined. Incidence: 1 in 2,000 Caucasian babies; less common in African-Americans, Hispanics, and Asians.

- **Toxoplasmosis:** Toxoplasmosis is a parasitic infection that can be transmitted through the mother's placenta to an unborn child. The disease-causing organism, which is found in uncooked or undercooked meat, can invade the brain, eye, and muscle, possibly resulting in blindness and mental retardation. The benefit of early detection and treatment is uncertain. Incidence: 1 in 1,000. But only one or two states screen for toxoplasmosis.

These aren't the only disorders that can be detected through newborn screening. Certain other rare disorders of body chemistry can also be detected. Other conditions that are candidates for newborn screening include the following:

- Duchenne muscular dystrophy, a childhood form of muscular dystrophy that can be detected through a blood test
- HIV (human immunodeficiency virus)
- Neuroblastoma, a type of cancer that can be detected with a urine test

Should I Request Additional Tests?

If you answer "yes" to any of the questions below, talk to your child's future doctor and perhaps a genetic counselor about requesting additional tests.

- Do you have a positive family history of an inherited disorder?

- Have you previously given birth to a child who's affected by a disorder?

- Did an infant in your family die because of a suspected metabolic disorder?

- Do you have another reason to believe that your child may be at risk for a certain condition?

> ♣ **It's A Fact!!**
> **Hearing Screening**
>
> Most, but not all states require newborns' hearing to be screened before they are discharged from the hospital. If your infant isn't examined at that time, it's important to make sure that he or she does get screened within the first three weeks of life. A child develops critical speaking and language skills in the first few years of life, and if a hearing loss is caught early, doctors can treat it so that it doesn't interfere with that development.

If your hospital can't or won't make expanded screening available to you, and your doctors believe additional testing would be worthwhile, you may want to contact outside laboratory services that provide supplemental testing for more than 30 metabolic disorders through a mail-order service available anywhere in the United States. The labs send out kits that are used to collect additional blood at the time of your baby's regular screening, and this sample is then mailed back for analysis. The cost ranges from $25 to $50.

How Is Newborn Screening Performed?

Within the first two or three days of life, your baby's heel will be pricked and a small sample of her blood will then be applied to a filter paper. Most states have identified a state or regional laboratory to which hospitals should send the samples for analysis. (If your hospital offers expanded screening that uses the new technology, your baby's sample may be sent to a private laboratory. Some states use a private lab for all of their studies.)

It's generally recommended that the sample be taken after the first 24 hours of life. Some tests, such as the one for PKU, may not be as sensitive if they're done too soon after birth. However, because mothers and newborns are often discharged within a day, some babies may be tested within the first 24 hours. If this happens, the AAP recommends that a repeat sample be taken no more than one to two weeks later. It's especially important that the

PKU screening test be run again for accurate results. Some states routinely do two tests on all infants.

Getting The Results

Different labs have different procedures for notifying families and pediatricians of the results. Some may send them to the hospital where your child was born and not directly to your child's doctor, which may mean a delay in getting the results to you. And although some states have a system that allows doctors to access the results via phone or computer, others may not. Ask your child's doctor how you will get the results and when you should expect them.

If a test result should come back abnormal, try not to panic. This does not necessarily mean that your child has the disorder in question. A screening test is not the same as a diagnostic test. The initial screening provides only preliminary information that must be followed up with more specific diagnostic testing.

If testing confirms that your child does have a disorder, your child's doctor may refer you to a specialist for further evaluation and treatment. Keep in mind that dietary restrictions and supplements, along with proper medical supervision, can often avert most of the serious physical and mental problems that were associated with metabolic disorders in the past.

You may also wonder whether the disorder can be passed on to any future children. This is a matter you'll want to discuss with your child's doctor and perhaps a genetic counselor. Also, if you have other children who weren't

✔ Quick Tip
Know Your Options

Because state programs are subject to change, you'll want to find up-to-date information about your state's (and individual hospital's) program. Talk to your child's doctor or contact your state's department of health for more information.

screened for the disorder, you may want to have this done. Again, talk this over with your children's doctor.

Chapter 48

Taking Care Of Your Newborn

Checkups And Shots

Checkups are a normal and important thing for babies. Even though your baby seems healthy, she should get checkups at one to two weeks of age, and at two, four, six, nine, and 12 months of age.

Ask your doctor for the results of the hearing screening if it was done in the hospital. If a hearing test was not done, ask your doctor for a referral for the test.

At each checkup, the doctor or nurse will do the following:

- examine your baby's head, eyes, ears, heart, lungs, and other body parts

- measure your baby's length, weight, and head size

- ask about your baby's hearing and vision

- ask you questions about how she eats, sleeps, and acts

- give you information about how a baby develops and grows

About This Chapter: Information in this chapter is excerpted from *Healthy Start, Grow Smart: Your Newborn*, U.S. Department of Education (www.ed.gov), 2002.

Your baby will be given shots (immunizations). Your baby will get her first shot in the hospital at birth. The shots help protect your baby from diseases such as hepatitis, measles, mumps, and chicken pox.

Some babies can get sick from the shots. Ask your doctor or nurse what signs to look for after your baby gets a shot so you will know if your baby needs medical care.

Keep a record or write down what happens at your baby's checkups. This record will help you and your doctor know about your baby's development and what is best for your baby.

✔ Quick Tip
When To Call The Baby's Doctor

One of the toughest and most nerve-racking things for new moms is figuring out when to call the doctor. If you suspect something is not right, you should always call the doctor. Even small changes in eating, sleeping, and crying can be signs of serious problems for newborns.

Call your pediatrician if your baby has any of the following symptoms:

- no urine in first 24 hours at home
- no bowel movement in the first 48 hours at home
- trouble breathing, very rapid breathing (more than 60 breaths per minute), or blue lips or fingernails
- pulling in of the ribs when breathing
- wheezing, grunting, or whistling sounds when breathing
- rectal temperature above 100.4° F or below 97.8° F
- persistent cough
- nosebleeds
- yellow or greenish mucus in the eyes
- pus or red skin at the base of the umbilical cord stump

Your Baby Should Sleep On Her Back

Most babies are healthy and have no problems when sleeping, but sometimes babies die in their sleep. This is called sudden infant death syndrome (SIDS), or crib death. Doctors have not found out what causes SIDS.

Research shows that babies who sleep on their backs are less likely to die from SIDS. However, if your baby has a health problem, your doctor may tell you to put her in another position.

Be sure your baby is sleeping on a firm mattress. Do not put your baby to sleep on soft or fluffy things such as a pillow, quilt, or waterbed. Keep stuffed animals out of the crib at sleep time.

- yellow color in whites of the eye and/or skin (jaundice) that gets worse 3 days after birth

- circumcision problems such as worrisome bleeding at the circumcision site, bloodstains on diaper or wound dressing larger than the size of a grape

- vomiting

- diarrhea (This can be hard to detect, especially in breastfed newborns. Diarrhea often has a foul smell and can be streaked with blood or mucus. Diarrhea is usually more watery or looser than normal. Any significant increase in the number or appearance of your newborn's regular bowel movements may suggest diarrhea.)

- fewer than six wet diapers in 24 hours

- a sunken soft spot (fontanel) on the baby's head

- refuses several feedings or eats poorly

- hard to waken or unusually sleepy

- extreme floppiness, lethargy, or jitters

- crying more than usual and very hard to console

Source: "When to Call the Baby's Doctor Print and Go Guide," National Women's Health Information Center, U.S. Department of Health and Human Services, January 2006.

Changing Baby's Diaper

Get everything you need before changing your baby's diaper. Once you start changing, do not take your eyes off your baby even for a second. They can get hurt or fall in an instant.

To change your baby's diaper do the following:

- Wash your hands before changing your newborn's diaper. Be sure to wash your hands with soap and water after each diaper change, too.

- Lay your baby on a clean surface. Take along a blanket or changing pad when you go out.

- Remove the dirty diaper.

- Use a washcloth dipped in clean, lukewarm water. Wash all the area on your baby that the diaper covers. Wipe from front to back to avoid infection.

- Every time you change a diaper, clean your baby's umbilical cord. Use a cotton swab that you have dipped in rubbing alcohol. Squeeze it so that it is almost dry. Gently clean off the sticky stuff around the cord where it touches your baby's tummy. The cord will fall off by itself in five to ten days. Your baby may cry when you touch the wet swab to the cord. Be gentle. Check with your doctor if your baby cries at other times when you touch the cord. Check with your doctor if the skin around the cord is red.

- Now put a clean diaper on your baby. If you are using pins, put your hand between the pin and your baby's skin. Do not let the diaper cover up the umbilical cord.

Newborns use about ten diapers every day. Change them as soon as they are wet. This can prevent rashes.

Preparing Your Baby's Bath

The following are things you should do when preparing to give your baby a bath:

- Get everything ready before you start the bath. This makes bathing your baby easier and safer.

- You can use your bathtub, kitchen sink, or a plastic baby tub. Use something to line the tub to keep your baby from slipping. If you use a foam liner for a tub, it needs to be dried out after each use. This prevents the growth of germs, or you can line the tub with a bath towel. Be sure to wash and dry it after each use.

- If you can, turn down your water heater to 120 degrees. Babies can get scalded easily. Fill the sink or tub with warm water. Always test the water with your wrist or elbow. The water should be comfortably warm but not hot.

- Keep mild soap, cotton balls, and a clean diaper in a shoe box or other container. Then you can bring the box in with the towel and washcloth to the room where you bathe your baby. When everything is ready, get your baby.

- If you forget an item, you will have to carry your baby with you.

- Never leave your baby alone in water. It is best not to answer the phone or the doorbell during your baby's bath. If you do, pick up your baby and carry her with you.

Bathing Your Baby

Give your baby a sponge bath until her umbilical cord or his circumcision, if any, is healed. After that, your baby can have a tub bath.

Use damp cotton balls to gently wipe your baby's eyes before you put her in the tub. Use a clean, damp washcloth, without soap, to wash her face. Gently wash the outside and back of each ear, and wash and dry under her neck.

Wash your baby's hair and scalp very gently, using soap or a baby shampoo. Do this only once or twice a week. Rinse with a damp cloth. Make sure that soapsuds do not get into her eyes. Wash her body, starting with the chest. After washing with a soapy washcloth, rinse the washcloth and rinse her off. Pat your baby dry with a bath towel.

Your newborn does not need to have a bath every day. Just clean her face, neck and diaper area whenever they are dirty.

Install Car Seats Carefully

Any time you take your baby anywhere in a car, put her in a car safety seat. This is best for your baby, and all states, the District of Columbia, Puerto Rico, and the U.S. Territories have child passenger safety laws.

Your baby will need different kinds of car safety seats as she grows. Right now, she should be in one that is made for a newborn baby. The safety seat should be placed in the back seat, facing the rear. Infants should never be placed in the front seat.

Make sure the car safety seat fits your car, is fastened in the car securely, and that the straps that go around your baby fit her snugly.

If you cannot afford a safety seat, the National Highway Traffic Safety Administration can provide information on resources that help low-income families purchase or borrow child car seats. You may call them at 888-327-4236 or visit their website at www.nhtsa.dot.gov.

Ways To Soothe Your Baby

Sometimes babies cry even when they have been fed, have clean diapers, and are healthy. Here are things you can try to find out what calms your baby down:

- Rock your baby in your arms or while sitting in a rocking chair.

- Stroke your baby's head very gently, or lightly pat her back or chest.

- Make soft noises, such as cooing, to let your baby know you are there and you care. Talk to your baby.

- Softly sing to your baby or play soft music.

- Wrap her up in a baby blanket (but not too tightly).

No matter how stressed you are, never shake your baby. Shaking your baby can cause blindness, brain damage, or even death.

✔ Quick Tip
Here is a simple tip to help your baby cry less—carry her. Research shows that babies who are carried more often do not cry as much as other babies.

Source: U.S. Department of Education, 2002.

Chapter 49

Questions And Answers About Breastfeeding

Why should I breastfeed?

Here are just some of the many good reasons why you should breastfeed your baby:

- Breast milk has just the right amount of fat, sugar, water, and protein that is needed for a baby's growth and development. Most babies find it easier to digest breast milk than they do formula.

- Breast milk has agents (called antibodies) in it to help protect infants from bacteria and viruses. Babies who are not exclusively breastfed for six months are more likely to develop a wide range of infections and diseases including ear infections, diarrhea, and respiratory illnesses. Infants who are not breastfed have a 21% higher postneonatal infant mortality rate in the U.S.

- Breastfed babies score higher on IQ tests in childhood, especially babies who were born prematurely.

- Nursing uses up extra calories, making it easier to lose the pounds of pregnancy. It also helps the uterus to get back to its original size and lessens any bleeding you might have after giving birth.

About This Chapter: Information in this chapter is from the National Women's Health Information Center, U.S. Department of Health and Human Services, May 2005.

- Breastfeeding lowers the risk of breast and ovarian cancers and possibly the risk of hip fractures and osteoporosis after menopause.

- Breastfeeding can help you bond with your baby.

How long should I breastfeed?

Babies should be fed with breast milk only, with no formula, for the first six months of life. The longer a mom and baby breastfeeds, the greater the benefits are for both mom and baby. Ideally, babies should receive breast milk through the first year of life, or for as long as both you and your baby wish. Solid foods can be added to your baby's diet, while you continue to breastfeed, when your baby is six months old. For at least the first six months, breastfed babies do not need supplements of water, juice, or other fluids. These can interfere with your milk supply if they are introduced during this time.

How do I know that my baby is getting enough milk from breastfeeding?

You can tell your baby is getting enough milk by keeping track of the number of wet and dirty diapers. In the first few days, when your milk is low in volume and high in nutrients, your baby will have only one or two wet diapers a day. After your milk supply has increased, your baby should have five to six wet diapers and three to four dirty diapers every day.

Is there any time when I should not breastfeed?

A few viruses can pass through breast milk. HIV (human immunodeficiency virus), the virus that causes AIDS, is one of them. If you are HIV positive, you should not breastfeed. If you have HIV and want to breastfeed, you can get breast milk for your baby from a milk bank.

Sometimes babies can be born with a condition called galactosemia, in which they cannot tolerate breast milk. This is because their bodies cannot break down the sugar galactose. Babies with classic galactosemia may have liver problems, malnutrition, or mental retardation. Since both human and animal milk contain the sugar lactose that splits into galactose and glucose, babies with classic galactosemia must be fed a special diet that is free of lactose and galactose.

✔ Quick Tip
Bottle Feeding

If you bottle feed your baby, ask your doctor what kind of formula is best for him. These are the three ways formula is sold:

• Powdered formula is the cheapest. You have to mix the powder with sterilized water.

• Concentrated formula is a liquid, but it is thick and must be mixed with sterilized water. It costs more than powdered formula.

• Ready-to-feed formula comes already mixed with water. It costs the most but is the easiest to use.

Follow formula mixing instructions carefully. There is a date on the formula. Do not use the formula after this date.

Wash reusable bottles made of plastic or glass. Also wash all equipment used to prepare formula. Use hot soapy water. Rinse the bottles in clean tap water. Then boil them five minutes in a covered pot or sterilizer.

To prepare formula, boil water for five minutes and cool it before mixing it with powdered or concentrated formula. If you are using bottles with disposable liners, throw away the liner after use. Store prepared formula in the refrigerator and use it within 48 hours.

Heat a bottle of formula by running hot water over it. Never heat formula in the microwave. It can get too hot. Check the temperature by shaking a few drops on your wrist. When it feels warm (not hot) on your wrist, it is cool enough to give to your baby.

When feeding your baby, hold his head a little higher than his tummy. Hold the bottom of the bottle up so that the nipple stays full of formula. This way, your baby does not swallow air and spit up. Never prop the bottle because your baby could choke. Always hold your baby while you feed him. Throw out any formula left in the bottle after a feeding.

Source: Excerpted from *Healthy Start, Grow Smart: Your Newborn*, U.S. Department of Education, 2002.

Mothers who have active, untreated TB (tuberculosis) or who are receiving any type of chemotherapy drugs should not breastfeed.

Some women think that when they are sick, they should not breastfeed; but most common illnesses, such as colds, flu, or diarrhea, cannot be passed through breast milk. In fact, if you are sick, your breast milk will have antibodies in it. These antibodies will help protect your baby from getting the same sickness.

Is it safe to take medications while breastfeeding?

Most medications pass into your milk in small amounts. If you take medication for a chronic condition such as high blood pressure, diabetes, or asthma, your medication may already have been studied in breastfeeding women, so you should be able to find information to help you make an informed decision with the help of your doctor. Newer medications and medications for rare disorders may have less information available.

Will breastfeeding tie me to my home?

Breastfeeding can be convenient no matter where you are because you do not have to bring along feeding equipment like bottles, water, or formula. Even if you want to breastfeed in private, you usually can find a woman's lounge or fitting room. If you want to go out without your baby, you can pump your milk beforehand and leave it for someone else to give your baby while you are gone.

How much do breastfeeding pumps cost, and what kind will I need?

Breast pumps range in price from under $50 (manual pumps) to over $200 (electrical pumps that include a carrying case and an insulated section for storing milk containers). If you are only going to be away from your baby a few hours a week, then you can purchase a manual pump, or one of the less expensive ones.

Part Seven

Teen Parenting Challenges

Chapter 50

Your Body After Pregnancy

Louise Kolin of New York City remembers clearly how she felt the first six weeks after delivering her baby. "I was very sore in my back and vaginal area. I felt like I had been beaten up." Although Louise's extreme physical condition was a result of a complicated delivery, all new mothers are met with varying degrees of physical challenges following childbirth and the weeks beyond.

Your body has performed a physical feat that far surpasses the demands expected of million-dollar athletes. In less than a year, you conceived, developed, and delivered a beautiful, living creature—a performance that used every ounce of your body's resources and then some.

Now your body must take on the rigorous new role of readjusting to its pre-pregnant state. "This is a time of incredible transition," says Gail Heathcote, CNM, MSN, CNS, and OB Outreach Coordinator at Spectrum Health-Downtown, in Grand Rapids, Michigan. Hormones continue to play a big role in directing your body through the necessary changes after childbirth. Progesterone and estrogen levels drop by 90 percent within the first few days after birth. This rapid plunge, plus the physical discomfort and fatigue, can wreak havoc on a new mother's emotional state—fluctuating from bouts of irritability to sustained periods of crying.

About This Chapter: Information in this chapter is from "Your Body After Pregnancy."
© 2003 American College of Nurse-Midwives. Reprinted with permission.

"The postpartum time is not exactly a time of bliss for most women. It is a time of incredible exhaustion," explains Heathcote. "A new mother needs to be treated like a princess for at least the first two weeks to make sure the family bonds. She also needs this time to get her energy back."

Fighting fatigue when your newborn does not sleep for more than two hours at a time may be impossible if mothers do not get help. "By day five or six, we see a crash where some new mothers get completely exhausted from lack of sleep," says Ruth Hope, CNM, MSN, of Birth Partners in Portland, Maine. "We have found that if mothers can get a good, solid four-hour pocket of sleep, they feel much better. That also combats depression and sleep deprivation."

✔ **Quick Tip**
Conquering Fatigue And Sleep Deprivation

Here are steps you can take to reduce, even eliminate, the number of days you feel groggy, irritable, and out of control:

- If breastfeeding, express your milk to allow your partner to share feeding the baby at night.

- Secure a friend to baby-sit while you nap during the day.

- Keep visitors at bay unless they have arrived to help.

- Minimize household chores—eat take-out, use paper plates, ignore clutter, and delegate dusting and vacuuming.

- Drink plenty of fluids.

- Steer clear of caffeine.

This certainly held true for Debbie Gray from Louisville, who recalls an easy adjustment to new motherhood. "I stayed with my mother for three months after Shelby was born while our house was being remodeled," she says. "I would take care of Shelby during the night and at 7 a.m. my mother would take over. I would get an extra hour-and-a-half of sleep. It was wonderful."

Within six weeks of delivery, your body is well on its way to recovery, and your midwife or doctor will want to check your progress. Although you may be anxious to return to your pre-pregnant shape, being informed of the process will help you to appreciate the phenomenal changes your body is undergoing and will help you to be more patient.

Abdomen: You may be surprised that your tummy still looks pregnant for a few weeks after delivery. Your uterus is still enlarged, and the muscles supporting it need time to become taut again. Within six weeks, in a process called involution, your uterus will contract back to its normal state, about the size of a small pear.

During involution, you will experience mild cramping, or after pains, that are instrumental in clamping off blood vessels and reducing postpartum bleeding. If you are breastfeeding, you may feel these after pains as your baby nurses since this activity stimulates oxytocin, the same hormone that causes the uterus to contract.

C-Section: If you delivered your baby via C-section, your recovery process will take longer, and you will need more help. You will need plenty of rest to recoup and will probably take pain pills that will make you groggy. As converse as it may sound, you will also need to keep moving to promote circulation and speed up the overall healing process.

✔ Quick Tip
On The Rebound

Once your baby arrives, it is easy to lose focus on your own recovery needs. These suggestions will help speed your recovery, both physically and mentally:

- **Tap Into Your Resources.** When friends and family want to help, say yes. Do not be shy about asking them to cook a meal, help with laundry, or watch the baby while you nap.

- **Rest.** Skip the superwoman routine and give yourself the time you need to recuperate.

- **Make Smart Food Choices.** Healthy eating will speed the healing process and boost your energy.

- **Get Fresh Air.** A 15–20 minute walk outdoors can restore your soul.

- **Establish A Routine.** You will regain your feelings of control.

- **Communicate With Your Partner About Everything.** Talk about things both physical and emotional.

- **Talk With Other New Moms.** You will discover secrets for coping that only these women can reveal.

Your incision should heal on the outside in two to three weeks but may remain sore and sensitive for up to two months. Some new moms contend with itching around the incision site for several months more.

Vagina: Your body's blood volume doubled during pregnancy. Now that it is no longer needed, the excess blood will be released through vaginal discharge, called lochia. For the first four or five days, the flow will be bright red and heavy, and may contain clots of blood. The color will gradually lighten and may change to yellowish-pink, then creamy white. The flow should taper off within two weeks. Occasionally, it may return to a reddish color, especially when breastfeeding. If the discharge becomes heavy, remains red in color, or has an unpleasant odor, contact your midwife or physician.

Other stored fluids are eliminated through your urine, which explains your seemingly endless trips to the bathroom. Some new mothers experience heavy perspiration—another way that your body chooses to eliminate excess fluids.

Perineum: The area between your vagina and rectum, the perineum, also takes time to heal, whether you receive stitches or not. The discomfort should not last more than four or five days. To provide relief and reduce the risk of infection, spray the area often using a peri-bottle filled with warm water. A warm bath or an ice pack will also relieve some of the discomfort.

Constipation: One of the more undesirable side effects of childbirth is constipation, which if not prevented, can affect new mothers for at least a few days, maybe even weeks. A number of factors are responsible for this sluggish intestinal behavior beginning with out-of-shape abdominal muscles, swollen tissue following delivery, use of anesthesia, epidurals, and some pain relievers. New mothers are also leery of putting pressure on the stitched perineal area and may inadvertently create a logjam.

There are several things you can do to lessen these problems: keep moving; do not sit for long periods of time; drink plenty of water; eat high-fiber foods, such as raw fruits and vegetables; and choose whole grains products.

Breasts: Your breasts have just spent nine months preparing themselves for nourishing your newborn. As they prepare for breastfeeding, they may

♣ It's A Fact!!
Healing Time

How quickly your body bounces back depends on a number of factors including your physical condition before and during pregnancy, difficulties during pregnancy and childbirth, and how well you take care of yourself in the weeks following delivery. If you experienced a normal delivery, here is a typical timetable you can expect:

- **Uterus:** 6 weeks to reach pre-pregnancy size, shape, and position

- **Lochia:** 4–6 weeks to completely stop

- **Episiotomy:** 4–5 days for pain to diminish, two weeks to heal

- **C-Section Incision:** 6–8 weeks for soreness to disappear

- **Weight Loss:** 10–12 pounds following delivery, 5–12 pounds in first few weeks

- **Sex:** normally six weeks to resume, unless your midwife or doctor tells you otherwise

feel achy, full, and tender to the touch. Your nipples may be sore. Wearing a supportive bra after childbirth, morning and night, will help protect the tender breast tissue and ease the achy feeling.

Eager for the job ahead, your breasts may fill themselves to overcapacity. Once engorged, they will feel rock hard and possibly hot to the touch. If your breasts are too full, your baby may have trouble latching on. Express a little milk manually or with a pump to soften the areola. Engorgement will occur less often once a feeding routine is established.

Skin: If your skin took on the proverbial glow of pregnancy, do not be alarmed when all of that changes after childbirth. Coupled with fatigue and a host of other physical changes, your skin may feel drier and less radiant. Rest assured, your skin will regain its normal tone once your menstrual cycle begins again.

Any skin discoloration that occurred during pregnancy, such as pregnancy mask or linea nigra, should disappear about three months after delivery. Eliminating sun exposure to these areas will keep the color from darkening. Stretch marks will also begin to fade.

Hair: If your hair is falling out at such a rate that baldness suddenly seems feasible, do not panic, the condition is only temporary. Prior to pregnancy, you probably lost an average of 100 hairs per day. Pregnancy hormones essentially put a hold on this hair loss rate, causing your locks to feel thicker and healthier. Now that hormone levels have drastically dropped, your hair must make up for lost time. All should be back to normal by the end of the baby's first year.

Exercise: You probably have not yet been given the green light to enter into a full-fledged exercise program (and mustering the energy to even think about it is unlikely right now), but starting with simple movements soon after childbirth will boost your energy and speed your recovery.

Begin with Kegel exercises as you did during pregnancy. These will help strengthen the pelvic floor, increase blood flow to the perineum, and promote healing. They will also help prevent incontinence and help your body to regain vaginal tone.

Walking is a perfect warm-up to more aerobic exercise later on. "Walk gently, 15 to 20 minutes per day, and get out into the fresh air," suggests Hope. "By eight weeks you should be ready to resume your regular exercise routine."

Nutrition: Watching what you eat for nine months may be a long enough sentence for some, but good nutrition is especially important now that your body is on the rebound. Careful food selection will help speed your physical recovery, keep your energy level up, and help with milk production. Unfortunately, with your new and demanding responsibilities, grabbing a quick bite may encourage unhealthy food choices. Eliminate this temptation by keeping cut-up fruit and veggies in the refrigerator for between meal munchies. Stock up on yogurt, low-fat cheese, and other quick fixes that offer essential body-healing nutrients.

Dieting to lose extra weight before your baby is weaned from breastfeeding could affect your milk supply. If you are not breastfeeding, your midwife or doctor may give you the thumbs up after your six-week visit. Remember, losing weight too quickly can slow the recovery process and lead to postpartum depression.

Sex: If you are like most new mothers, it may take a while for your desire for sex to return. There is good reason. Your hormones are still at work; you may be experiencing perineal tenderness, vaginal dryness and fatigue; and your thoughts are preoccupied with caring for your baby. "Most women say they are never having intercourse again, and certainly not by six weeks," declares Heathcote. However, she finds that the majority has resumed sex by their six-week checkup.

Waiting six weeks after delivery to resume intercourse will allow your uterus to heal and reduce the risk of infection. However, depending on the type of labor you had, this time frame may be altered.

Contraception: Since ovulation occurs about two weeks before your period returns, it is especially important to use birth control each time you and your partner have sex. The most commonly recommended form of contraception during this six-week time frame is the condom used in conjunction with spermicidal jelly, but consult with your midwife or doctor for alternate suggestions.

Your midwife or doctor will typically schedule you for a six-week checkup after delivery. By this time, your body is on the mend, and you have had time to adjust, though not fully, to your new lifestyle. Any concerns, both physical and emotional, should be discussed now, if not sooner.

The physical examination will include checks of the following:

- shape, size, and location of uterus to insure that it has returned to its pre-pregnant state
- episiotomy or C-section stitches have healed
- vaginal discharge is clear
- blood pressure
- weight—down by about 20 pounds since before delivery
- cervix, vagina, ovaries, fallopian tubes, and perineum
- abdominal wall if you had a C-section
- breasts
- hemorrhoids
- birth control
- urine sample

- legs for swelling or varicose veins

- Pap test

You will be encouraged to discuss parenting issues, social support, sex, birth control, exercise, diet, breastfeeding, and emotional concerns. Prior to your visit, write down questions of concern so that you will not forget them.

Chapter 51

Baby Proofing Your Home

Babies learn quickly in their first year. For new parents, it's a pleasant surprise to see how soon they begin moving and exploring. But turn your back for a moment, and the infant who was squirming helplessly on a blanket is suddenly crawling across the room at high speeds.

Children are naturally curious. Tasting, touching, and feeling are how infants and toddlers learn about the world around them. Take a moment to look at your surroundings from a youngster's point of view. Then make any necessary adjustments to baby proof your home.

Suffocation And Choking

• Infants, when placed on an adult bed of any kind, can roll into the space between the wall and the mattress and suffocate. Exercise caution if sleeping in the same bed with an infant. It is possible for an infant to become wedged between your body and the mattress and suffocate. Infants should never be placed on top of soft surfaces like sofas, large soft toys, sofa cushions, pillows, and waterbeds, or on top of blankets, quilts, or comforters.

About This Chapter: Information in this chapter is from "Baby-proofing Your Home," a fact sheet produced by the National Safety Council, © 2004. Reprinted with permission. For more information, visit the website of the National Safety Council at www.nsc.org.

- Babies should sleep on their backs.

- Crib bars should be no more than 2 3/8 inches apart to prevent infants from getting their heads stuck between them. Cribs manufactured after 1974 must meet this and other strict safety standards.

- The crib mattress must fit tightly so there are no gaps for an infant to fall into. Keep the crib clear of plastic sheets, pillows, and large stuffed animals or toys. These can be suffocation hazards.

♣ **It's A Fact!!**

Mechanical suffocation and suffocation by ingested objects cause the most home fatalities to children 0–4 years of age. Drownings and home fires also contribute to the death of young children.

- Keep toys with long strings or cords away from infants and young children. A cord can become wrapped around an infant's neck and cause strangulation. Toys with long strings, cords, loops, or ribbons should never be hung in cribs or playpens. Similarly, pacifiers should never be attached to strings or ribbons around the baby's neck.

- Place an infant or child's bed away from any windows. Check window coverings for potentially hazardous pull cords.

- Use child safety gates at the top and bottom of all staircases and be sure they're installed correctly. Avoid accordion-style safety gates with large openings that children could fit their heads through.

- Choking is a common cause of unintentional death in children under the age of 1. Avoid all foods that could lodge in a child's throat. Some examples include popcorn, grapes, foods with pits, raisins, nuts, hard candies, raw vegetables, and small pieces of hotdogs.

- Never let children of any age eat or suck on anything, such as hard candy, while lying down.

- Keep floors, tables, and cabinet tops free of small objects that could be swallowed. Such objects include coins, button-sized batteries, rings, nails, tacks, and broken or deflated balloons.

Falls And Burns

- A mixer faucet on the basin, tub, and shower will prevent scalds. Set your hot water thermostat for 120° F. A baby's bath water should be 100°F. Always check bath water temperature with your wrist or elbow before putting a baby in to bathe. Don't allow children in a whirlpool, Jacuzzi, or hot tub. Their bodies are more sensitive to hot water.

- Teach youngsters that matches are tools for adults, not toys. Adults should never ignite lighters or matches in front of children. Store matches in a fire-resistant container out of the reach of youngsters.

- Do not smoke, use matches, or drink hot beverages while holding an infant. Don't leave burning cigarettes unattended.

- Remember that radiators, heating vents, space heaters, fireplaces, stoves, and hot water taps are not always hot. Children can touch them once safely and the next time receive a severe burn.

- Keep electrical cords and wires out of the way so toddlers can't pull, trip, or chew on them. Cover wall outlets with safety caps.

Drowning

- Never leave a child unsupervised in the bathtub. If you must leave the room for a telephone call or to answer the door, wrap the child in a towel and take him or her with you. Don't leave a small child alone with any container of liquid, including wading pools, scrub buckets, and toilets.

- A swimming pool drowning could also be called a "silent death" as there is rarely a splash or cry for help to alert parents to the problem. The typical drowning victim is a boy between 1 and 3 years old who is thought not to be in the pool area at the time of the incident.

    - Fence in the pool completely. Doors leading to the pool area should be self-closing and self-latching or equipped with exit alarms and should never be propped open.

- Never take your eyes off children when they are in or near any body of water, not even for a second. Don't rely on inflatable devices, such as inner tubes, water wings, inflatable mattresses and toys, or other similar objects to keep a youngster afloat. Keep toys, tricycles, and other playthings away from the pool area. A toddler near the water could unexpectedly fall in.

- All pool owners and their families are encouraged to seek training in swimming, lifesaving, first aid, and cardiopulmonary resuscitation.

If it seems that there is a lot to do before that new bundle of joy comes home, you are correct. However, simple safety checks can help ensure that you and baby will have many happy and healthy years together.

Chapter 52

Child Care

Using A Babysitter

Safety/First Aid

- Ask if the babysitter knows infant/child CPR (cardiopulmonary re-suscitation) and Rescue Breathing.

- Remind the babysitter that infants should not be placed on an adult bed of any kind.

- Remind the babysitter to place the baby on his or her back to sleep.

- Be sure that the babysitter knows the signs of illness in an infant including changes in skin color, sweating, nausea or vomiting, and diarrhea.

- Show the babysitter where the fire extinguishers are kept and explain how they are used.

About This Chapter: Information under the headings "Using A Babysitter" and "Choosing A Child Care Provider" are excerpted from "Childcare/Babysitters" and "Child Care Provider Checklist," National Women's Health Information Center, U.S. Department of Health and Human Services, January 2006. Additional text from Child Care Aware is cited separately within the chapter.

- Be sure to show the babysitter where the first aid supplies are kept.

- Remind the babysitter to keep all balloons or plastic items away from the baby.

- Instruct the babysitter that children should never be unsupervised in the bathtub.

- He/she should take them with him/her if they must answer the telephone or the doorbell.

- Remind the babysitter to keep the bathroom door closed and the toilet seat and lid down when not in use.

Familiarity With Your House

- Before leaving be sure to give the babysitter a tour of the house.

- Ensure that all windows have been closed and that the babysitter knows to keep them closed.

- Show the babysitter how to operate your child safety gates and indicate where they need to be kept.

- Show the babysitter where the flashlights are located.

- Make sure that you have put away all sharp items including scissors, knives, and any other objects that can cause injury.

Choosing A Child Care Provider

Steps To Choosing Quality Child Care

- Visit several child care homes or centers. Visit the home or center more than once and stay as long as possible so you can get a good feel for what the care will be like for your child. Continue to visit even after you start using the home or center.

- Make sure the place is cheerful and not too quiet, which can mean not enough activity.

- Count the number of children in the group and the number of staff members caring for them. The fewer the number of children for each staff member, the more attention your child will get.

- Ask about the background and experience of all staff that will have contact with your child in the home or center.

- Find out more about efforts in your community to improve the quality of child care. Ask if the home or center is involved in these activities. Consider getting yourself involved.

Things To Consider When Choosing A Child Care Provider

Here is some important information to measure the quality of a child care provider or center.

The Caregivers/Teachers: Are children greeted when they arrive and are their needs met quickly even when things get busy? Do the caregivers/teachers have training in CPR, first aid, and early childhood education and are they involved in continuing education programs for themselves? Will the caregivers/teachers always be available to answer your questions and deal with your concerns? Are parent's ideas welcomed and are there ways for you to get involved?

The Setting: Is the atmosphere bright and pleasant? Is there a fenced-in outdoor play area with a variety of safe equipment and can the caregivers/teachers see the entire playground at all times? Are there different areas for resting, quiet play, and active play and is there enough space for the children in all of these areas?

The Activities: Is there a daily balance of play/activity time, story time, and rest time? Are the activities right for each age group? Are there enough toys and learning materials for the number of children and are the toys clean, safe, and within reach of the children?

In General: Do you agree with the discipline practices? Do you hear the sounds of happy children? Are children comforted when needed? Is the program licensed or regulated? Are surprise visits by parents encouraged? Will your child be happy there?

♣ It's A Fact!!
Child Care Programs
Help Teen Parents Stay In School

Years ago, long before she started high school, Kate—a bright, talkative over-achiever with a knack for everything from basketball to math—had a vision of her future. In it she saw a varsity athlete, a straight A student, a college scholarship, and a career in either medicine or biotechnology. It would be simple, she thought: Work hard and the rest will fall into place. "Was I naïve," she recalls. "Little did I know."

Following a brief fling with an older student, Kate became pregnant her sophomore year in high school. "I was 15," says Kate. "I had no idea what I was getting into."

Kate decided to continue the pregnancy and have the child, and that summer she became the mother of a brand new baby boy. At the time she was excited, but quite understandably, she was also terrified. "I didn't know what to do," she says. "I couldn't leave school. It would be the end of my life. My parents couldn't help. I was in serious trouble."

Torn Between Two Worlds

Kate, who has since resolved her crisis with the help of relatives, friends, and a local low-cost child care service, is among the thousands of U.S. high school students who become parents every year. Kate was lucky—her son is healthy, and now she's even looking at colleges.

But not all teen parents are this fortunate. Faced with the daunting task of juggling the challenges of parenting with the obligations of school, many teen parents, in desperation, drop out—a move that can undermine their future financial success and personal fulfillment. But their children need them, and they can't afford to pay for professional child care. As far as they know, they have no choice.

Helping Out

For many teen parents, however, help is available; they just have to know where to find it. Thanks to the Child Care and Development Block Grant (CCDBG), a child care services funding program administered by the U.S. Department of Health and Human Services, many states provide money to teenage parents who need it to be able to afford child care so they can stay in school.

Various other state-, county-, and city-based programs provide similar child care funds or services for teenage parents. In New York City, for example, the Living for the Young Family through Education (LYFE) program is a school-based service providing free child care during the school day in at least 40 different schools. Just a short drive north, the Massachusetts Department of Early Education and Care oversees that state's Teen Parent Child Care program (TPCC), which helps teen parents find free child care, transportation to and from child care services, and other parent-friendly resources.

Elsewhere, in Alexandria, VA, the city-subsidized Early Childhood Development program offers teenage parents similar help; and at the Teen Parent Project in Cook County, IL, teens are eligible for free child care support and other services while they attend school.

Teen Parent Project spokesperson, Valicia Johnson, says many of the teens they serve have nowhere else to turn. "We find child care services in their neighborhood and help them find ways to pay for it," says Johnson. "We also have a job referral program that helps them find jobs near school or home; and we work with them to see if they qualify for food stamp benefits and low-cost medical care."

Where To Go

Depending on where you live, there may be low-cost child care services available in your area, too. To find out, the following national programs are a good place to start:

- **Child Care Aware** (1-800-424-2246): Call this service for the name and number of your local Child Care Resource and Referral (CCR&R) agency. The website includes a search engine that uses your zip code to find your local agency (http://www.childcareaware.org).

- **National Child Care Information Center** (1-800-616-2242): A program of the U.S. Department of Health and Human Services Administration for Children and Families, the center maintains a list of state and regional offices providing information on local subsidized child care services (http://www.nccic.org).

- **Head Start**: Another program of the U.S. Department of Health and Human Services, Head Start provides education and early childhood development services for low-income families with children ages five and younger. Use the website's search engine to find Head Start services in your area (http://www.acf.hhs.gov/programs/hsb).

Source: Reprinted with permission from Planned Parenthood® Federation of America, Inc. © 2007 PPFA. All rights reserved. For additional information, visit www.plannedparenthood.org.

Choosing A Relative As A Caregiver

Text under this heading is from "All In The Family: Making Child Care Provided By Relatives Work For Your Family," 2001. Reprinted with permission from Child Care Aware, a program of NACCRRA. Childcareaware.org 1-800-424-2246, 2001.

Why Parents Often Choose A Relative Caregiver

- Comfort—because children are generally more at ease with people they know.

- Love and attention—if it's a close family member who has a genuine affection for your child.

- Trust—because you know them well and you know what values you share.

- Flexibility to meet your schedule, especially if it is part-time, evening hours, or rotating shifts.

- Familiar location in your or a relative's home.

There Can Also Be Problems

- Relative care can be lonely for the child and your relative.

- Child care raises unexpected and sensitive issues that can complicate family relationships.

- You and your relative may underestimate how time consuming and tiring it is to provide child care.

- Ideas about discipline may differ.

- Children's needs change as they grow, and you may need to change child care arrangements.

Making It Work Smoothly For Everyone

- Take time to talk regularly, when children are not around.

- Discuss and clarify your ideas about discipline and how you want your relative to set rules and guide your child.

- Talk about your child's daily routines: sleep, crying, feeding, and outdoor play.

- Make sure your relative has the time, energy, and health to keep up with your child.

- Ask if your relative sees this as a long-term or short-term arrangement.

- Discuss plans with your relative about television, reading, friends, and chores for your child.

Remember, Safety First

- Double check for child safety in your or a relative's home. Use a safety checklist.

- Prepare for emergencies with a safety plan, a fire extinguisher, medical and allergy information, and a list of work, fire, and emergency phone numbers.

- Agree on who may pick up your child.

- Remember, safety for a young child means no hitting or shaking.

Paying A Relative For Child Care Should Be In An Agreement

- Be clear about exactly when and how you'll pay your family member.

- Write down your agreement so there is no misunderstanding about your arrangements and payments.

- You'll need to agree about holidays, vacations, and sick days for your child or relative.

- Be creative. In addition to money, what can you do to show your appreciation?

- Learn about sample agreements and tax implications from your local child care resource and referral agency.

Families Are Forever: Keeping Good Relationships

- Offer to pay for a first aid and CPR class.

- Ask your family member what might be helpful to them in doing child care.

- Call your child care resource and referral agency to see what information is available for relative caregivers. Ask about resources like toy libraries, story hours, and community activities.

- If you change child care, remember, your relative caregiver is still family.

When There Are Problems

- Find the right time and place to talk about it, when you are both relaxed.

- Express gratitude for all your family does for your child.

- Keep the focus on the child.

- Show respect for your relative's point of view, even when you disagree.

- Think about how to avoid the problem in the future.

- Decide if you are still comfortable with the arrangements or if you will need to start looking for other child care.

You May Need To Make A Change

- If your relative finds it too hard to take care of your child everyday.

- When your child needs a preschool experience with other children.

- If your schedule changes.

- If it just doesn't work out.

But Family Is Still Family

- Thank your relative for helping.

- Consider asking if your relative could help with backup care.

Chapter 53

Are You Considering Emancipation?

Emancipation is a legal process by which minors can attain legal adulthood before reaching the age at which they would normally be considered adults. The status of emancipation can mean different things in different circumstances. For example, being emancipated for the purpose of public assistance requires criteria that are different than those required of a minor who seeks emancipation in the eyes of the law in general. The legal status of emancipation generally gives to minors rights that are similar to adults and makes a difference in the acquisition of health care and housing, for example. This chapter outlines some of the major issues concerning emancipation.

What does emancipation mean?

Emancipation refers to the release of a minor from parental control. Courts generally say that deciding whether a minor can claim an emancipated status is a question of fact. This means that a judge will look at all of the applicant's circumstances to determine whether the minor is free from parental control and able to live on her own as an adult. A judge will usually consider the following factors: age, marital status, ability to be self-supportive, and desire to live independently of parents. The court will consider whether the minor is employed and has a stable source of income as well as a place to live.

About This Chapter: Information in this chapter is from "Emancipation," © 2007 Juvenile Law Center. All rights reserved. Reprinted with permission.

Emancipation does not mean being treated like an adult in all situations. For example, emancipated minors cannot vote or drink alcoholic beverages. Further, emancipated minors' signatures on contracts (like leases) are not binding in the same way as those of adults. In addition, a minor who is, or has been pregnant, acquires rights similar to adults with respect to their own children. As long as a minor mother cares for her child adequately, she has the same rights as any other parent.

The status of emancipation also frees parents of responsibilities to their minor children. Parents, for example, do have an obligation to provide financial support for their children to the best of their abilities. This obligation would no longer exist if the minor becomes emancipated.

Is it lawful for a minor who has not yet been emancipated to live on her own or with an adult friend or relative that does not have legal custody of the minor?

Yes. Parents can allow their children to live on their own or with other adults as long as the health or safety of the minor is not endangered. This, however, does not mean that the minor is emancipated. In these situations, the parent or legal guardian will ultimately be legally responsible for the minor if she or he does not live with them. For example, parents or guardians will still be responsible for their child's welfare and for any truancy from school.

What are the consequences of a minor moving away from the parents' home without their permission?

If a minor moves away from the home of his or her parents or legal guardians without their permission, that minor can be picked up by authorities as a runaway or could be placed through Children and Youth Services and found dependent by the court. The minor might be found dependent on the grounds that the parents were not able to control the minor.

Is a parent responsible for the acts of a child who no longer lives at home?

In most cases, parents are responsible for the acts of an unemancipated minor who does not live in their home. This means, for example, that if a minor is charged with an offense in juvenile court and is fined, his or her parents would be ultimately responsible for the fine. Parents will not be held responsible for such acts if the minor is emancipated. Parents can attempt to argue that the minor is, in effect, emancipated and provide adequate documentation of that status if they want to avoid responsibility for the acts of their child. A parent, however, cannot avoid liability by deserting a minor.

Is emancipation a permanent status?

No. A minor remains emancipated only as long as he or she remains financially independent of his or her parents, is free of their care and control, and living independently. If, before turning eighteen, a minor moves back in with her parents or is supported by them, she is no longer considered emancipated.

Does getting married automatically lead to emancipation?

No. Marriage itself does not emancipate a minor for all purposes. Marriage is one factor among the minor's whole situation that a judge will consider when determining whether the minor should be emancipated. Usually the fact that a minor is married demonstrates that he is independent of his parents; but there are some cases where this is not so, and therefore the court must consider other factors in addition to marital status to determine whether the minor is living independently and is self-supportive. When married couples live away from parents and support themselves, they satisfy the general standard of emancipation. If minors divorce or obtain an annulment, however, they can revert to unemancipated status.

Marriage does satisfy the definition of emancipation contained in the public assistance regulations. In addition, married minors can consent to their own medical, dental, and health care.

Teens considering marriage should know that individuals under the age of eighteen need parental consent to get married. Minors under the age of sixteen need the consent of a judge as well as parental consent to get married.

Does becoming a parent automatically lead to emancipation?

Teenagers do acquire some of the rights of adults when they have a child. For example, teenage parents have the right to custody of their child and to make decisions regarding the child's upbringing, such as consenting to medical treatment, educational planning, and adoption. Teenage parents maintain these rights regardless of whether they live with their own parents or not, as long as they adequately care for their child. Teenage mothers also have the right to consent to their own health care, except for abortions.

♣ It's A Fact!!
Becoming a parent does not emancipate a minor for all purposes. If a minor is not able to support herself and does not live independently of her parents, she is not considered emancipated, whether or not she has a child.

Who decides whether a minor can be emancipated?

When a petition for emancipation is filed with the court, a judge will decide whether the minor should be emancipated. In these cases, the judge can issue a court decree, and the minor can get a copy for his or her records to prove his or her status. In addition, particular authorities can treat a minor as emancipated in certain situations. These authorities have their own procedures for determining when to work with minors without parental involvement. These procedures do not have the same all-encompassing effect as a judicial decree. For instance, school districts generally make their own decisions about who is emancipated for the purpose of attending school. Their decision to treat a minor as emancipated, however, will be only for the purpose of school; it will not necessarily extend to other areas and does not have the same effect as a judicial decree. Additionally, a local housing authority may require that a minor who seeks public housing present a court decree of emancipation as a condition of eligibility.

What is emancipation for the purpose of schooling?

Minors can be emancipated for the purposes of schooling. Emancipation is usually requested by minors when they are living away from their parents, are not placed with an approved guardian, and want to attend school in an area in which their parents do not live. Emancipation may be necessary in these cases because students under the age of twenty-one are entitled to attend public school but only in the district in which their parents live.

Emancipation enables minors to attend school in the area where they are living. Emancipation for school purposes is only for school purposes and does not carry with it any other rights. Similarly, a minor may not need to meet the requirements for emancipation in general (such as being self-supportive) to become emancipated for school purposes.

Most school districts make their own decisions about whether children are emancipated for the purposes of establishing residency within a school district and of assuming responsibility for school absences (parents will no longer be responsible for the child's truancy). Schools tend to base their decisions on whether the child lives with her parents and if she receives any support from her parents.

When a minor wants a school district to rule that she is emancipated, she can help her case by having her parents or legal guardians send a letter to the school district stating that the child does not live with the parents, that the parents do not provide financial support, and/or that both the parents and the child agree that the child should be emancipated.

What is emancipation for the purpose of public assistance?

Caseworkers at public assistance offices make the initial determination of whether a minor is emancipated for the purpose of receiving general assistance and Temporary Assistance to Needy Families (TANF). However, if there is a dispute about eligibility, a fair hearing may be conducted by the Department of Public Welfare, and a decision about the minor's status will be made by a hearing examiner. A minor will not go before a judge in court to determine whether she is emancipated for the purpose of public assistance and will not receive a judicial decree that says she is emancipated.

♣ **It's A Fact!!**

Being emancipated for the purpose of public assistance can serve as proof of the child's independent status; however, it does not mean that a minor will be considered emancipated for all purposes, because filing a general assistance application means that the applicant is not able to support him or herself.

What is general assistance?

To be eligible for general assistance benefits, a person who is sixteen or older and under twenty-one must meet the following criteria to establish that he or she is emancipated for the purpose of receiving these benefits. To prove emancipation a minor needs to meet one of the following criteria:

1. The minor must have left the parental household and have his own residence established independent of parental control. (If the minor returns to live with his parents, he will no longer be considered emancipated unless he remains independent of his parent's control.)

2. The minor must be married. If the minor is married, it does not matter whether the minor continues to live in the parental household. If this marriage is terminated by death or divorce, the minor will stay emancipated. However, if the marriage ends by annulment, that minor will no longer be considered emancipated. If a minor meets the above criteria for emancipation, he or she will be able to complete an application for general assistance. An emancipated minor will still need to meet the other eligibility requirements for general assistance, but the emancipated status allows the minor to proceed with his or her application as if he or she was an adult.

An unmarried child committed to the care and control of a county agency (like Department of Human Services) can become emancipated before the age of eighteen only by the action of the court.

There are certain limited situations in which an unemancipated minor may receive general assistance.

What is Temporary Assistance to Needy Families (TANF)?

Since the welfare system has been reformed, Aid to Families with Dependent Children (AFDC) no longer exists. The new welfare law is called Temporary Assistance to Needy Families (TANF) and has added several requirements for receipt of aid that differ from those of AFDC, which affects the minor's qualifications for emancipation.

This law requires that minor parents or pregnant minors must live with a parent, guardian, or adult relative or caretaker to receive TANF benefits. A

✦ It's A Fact!!

The federal law allows states to put a cap on the number of children for which a mother may be allowed to collect benefits under TANF, and this is true regardless of whether the mother is emancipated or not.

minor parent also must be enrolled in school or employed to receive benefits. By federal law, however, a minor parent with children under the age of six cannot be penalized if she cannot meet the work or employment requirement due to lack of child care.

This chapter is provided for informational purposes only and does not constitute legal advice. Applicability of the legal principles discussed in this chapter may differ substantially in individual situations, different counties, or in different states. If you have a specific concern or legal problem, do not rely on this chapter. Be sure to seek the advice of an attorney about your particular situation and facts.

Chapter 54

Finding A Place To Live

Living With Your Parents

Can my parents make me leave home because I am pregnant or have a child?

If you are a minor child, your parents must provide shelter for you. It is against the law for your parents to "kick you out" so that you have to find your own shelter or sleep outside. This does not mean that your parents must let you live in their home, however. They may provide shelter for you in their home, or they may arrange for you to stay somewhere else (as long as the place meets basic needs). Examples of places where your parents could arrange for you to stay are:

- with a relative or a family friend,

- in a boarding school,

- in a maternity home, or

About This Chapter: Information in this chapter is from *Pregnancy and Parenting: A Legal Guide for Adolescents, Second Edition.* © 2006 University of North Carolina at Chapel Hill. Reprinted with permission. Note: "A Place to Live" reflects federal and North Carolina law only. Most states have law on the points mentioned in the section and those laws vary. To see the document from which this excerpt was taken and three other legal guides on minors' pregnancy and parenting, go to http://www.teenpregnancy.unc.edu.

- in some other place where treatment is provided (such as a hospital or a group home).

✤ It's A Fact!!

Your pregnancy or the birth of your child does not change your parents' legal duty to care for and supervise you.

Your pregnancy or the birth of your child does not change your parents' legal duty to care for and supervise you. If they fail to meet this duty, the Department of Social Services (DSS) can ask a court to find that you are neglected. Your parents do not have to house their grandchildren, though. Under the law, as long as you are an unemancipated minor child, you are expected to live where your parent or guardian tells you to live.

What if I want to leave my parent's home?

Experts believe that, in most cases, it is better for a teen mother to live at home with her parents after her baby is born. This belief is based on studies showing that young mothers who live with their parents are more likely to finish high school (possibly because live-at-home teen mothers receive more encouragement and/or more help with child care).

Because of this belief that home is usually the best place, many laws and funding programs try to encourage young mothers to stay at home. For example, leaving your parent's home may keep you from getting money from the government (Temporary Assistance to Needy Families [TANF]) to help support your child.

Must a minor parent always live in a parent's home to get cash assistance (TANF)?

Not always. There are two exceptions to this rule. You do not have to live at home if:

- you are a teen parent who is married or emancipated, or

- living in your parent's home puts you or your child's physical or emotional health at risk.

If you cannot live at home because physical or emotional harm might come to you or your child, the Department of Social Services (DSS) must help you find a suitable, adult-supervised place to live. If you think you or your child might be at risk in your parent's home, call DSS and ask for the Child Protective Services section. Tell them that you are reporting your situation and ask them to investigate. They must tell you whether they will investigate, and if they do look into your situation, they must tell you what they decide.

Where can I live besides my parent's home?

Sometimes a minor mother moves out of her parent's home with no plan for where she and her baby will stay. The young mother may then try living with a series of relatives and friends, but this may not be good for her or her child. If you are moving from place to place, it is very hard to stay in school, to find and keep a job, and to keep up with appointments for your child and yourself, including appointments that keep you eligible for benefits such as Medicaid and TANF. It is even hard to keep up with your mail. For those reasons and perhaps more, you need an adult to help you if you have been asked to leave home or have decided to leave on your own and have no place to stay where your needs will be met. (If you are living with a man you are not married to, the Department of Social Services (DSS) will not consider you to be living in an appropriate adult-supervised arrangement.) If you do not know an adult who can help you, try to find one at school, the police or sheriff's department, the health department, the Department of Social Services, a recreation center, or at a church, synagogue, or mosque. Look for places that show the yellow sign that says "Safe Place." The adults in places with these signs will call someone to meet with you and help you make a plan for yourself and your child.

✤ It's A Fact!!

Under federal law, an unmarried parent who is 17 or younger and has custody of a child older than 12 weeks must be in school or involved in another educational activity and must live at home or in an approved, adult-supervised setting in order to receive government assistance.

Can my parents keep my child while making me live elsewhere?

Your parents may not keep your child (their grandchild) while you are forced to live somewhere else, except in the following situations:

- You are in detention, jail, or prison.

- You are in a hospital or other treatment place and cannot care for the child.

- The Department of Social Services and/or court has given them custody of their grandchild (your child).

Renting Your Own Apartment, House, Or Mobile Home (Trailer)

Can I rent a place for myself?

Probably not. Owners and rental agents for apartments, houses, and mobile homes usually will not sign leases with minors. Also, utility companies that provide water, electricity, natural gas, and heating oil usually will not start these services in a minor's name. This is because, under the law, a minor is not responsible for a contract that he or she signs. So, even if you signed a lease for housing, the landlord probably could not collect the rent money if you did not pay.

You may have an adult relative or friend who is willing to sign a lease for you so that you can have your own place. If so, the adult is listed as the person renting the apartment, house, or trailer. He or she is the tenant, which makes him or her legally responsible for the rent and for paying for damage to the property. You and your child are listed as occupants. An adult who signed for your apartment, house, or trailer would be taking on a big responsibility, and it is important for you to know that. It is also important for you to understand a few laws and legal definitions about renting a place to live.

What is a lease?

A lease is a contract or legally enforceable agreement between a landlord (the owner of the property) and a tenant (the person who is renting the property). In the lease, the landlord and tenant agree on the rules for the rental of the property. Once the landlord and tenant both sign the lease, they are required to do what the lease says (unless the lease says something that is illegal under the landlord-tenant laws).

Rental leases can be either written or spoken, depending on how long the landlord and tenant agree the lease will last. It is usually much better to have a lease in writing. That way, everyone is clear about his or her responsibilities under the lease, and many misunderstandings can be avoided.

What should be in a lease?

These are important things you should look for in a lease:

- the address of the property being rented
- the name and address of the landlord
- how much the rent is per week or month
- how much the deposit is and how you can get it back (A deposit is money that a tenant gives a landlord before moving in, which the landlord can use to pay for damage the tenant might do to the housing unit.)
- exactly when rent must be paid
- how long you are renting for (This is called the "term of the lease"—for example, some leases require the tenant to rent the property for six months or a year, while other leases only call for renting one month at a time.)
- how the tenant and landlord must notify each other about ending the lease

A lease should also make clear whether the tenant or landlord must pay the utility bills and how the property is to be maintained. Some leases also say whom, or at least how many people, may live in the house, apartment, or mobile home. The adult who helps you rent a place to live will be violating the lease if the lease names who may live in the house or apartment and you and your child are not named.

What are a landlord's and a tenant's main duties?

The tenant (or a responsible adult if the tenant is a minor) must pay the rent and not damage the property. In return, the landlord must keep the property in a reasonable condition. If your community has a minimum housing code (rules about health and safety in housing), then the landlord must follow that code. If the landlord does not make necessary repairs after you inform him of the problem and you believe that your health or safety is at risk, you should report the situation to your local housing office. It is illegal for your landlord to take action against you by, for example, increasing the rent or trying to evict you, because you or the person signing the lease reported the poor condition of the property.

Can I be put out of an apartment before the lease is up?

If the rent is not paid on time, a landlord may try to have a tenant put out (evicted). Some landlords try to use methods that are illegal. A landlord may not try to make you leave by hassling you, locking you out, putting your things in the street, or turning off the electricity, gas, water, or other essential services. Instead, the law says that unless the lease says otherwise, the landlord must notify the tenant to pay the rent or else the rental agreement will be over.

Public Assistance For Housing

Can I get public assistance for housing?

You may know that some people in your community get government assistance in buying or renting a home, and you may want similar assistance to rent an apartment. Once you are 18 you may be able to get public assistance for housing. However, most public housing authorities have rules that stop you from even getting on a waiting list for an apartment or for rental assistance until your 18th birthday. And even then, you are not guaranteed housing assistance.

In the United States, there is no legal right to safe, decent, and affordable housing. Instead, housing assistance is seen as a benefit that the government may provide. In recent years, the federal government has set aside little money for housing assistance. As a result, many public housing agencies have cut back the number of people they serve.

What should I do if I'm homeless?

Many cities and towns have homeless shelters. The law allows minors to use emergency shelters for the homeless without their parent's permission. However, if the shelter staff let you stay, they will contact your parents within a day or so. Some shelters will take a minor mother with her child, but unfortunately, quite a few will not. To find out if there is a shelter where you are, call the police or the Department of Social Services (DSS).

The National Runaway Switchboard:

- takes calls from anyone, 24 hours a day, every day of the year
- keeps calls confidential (NRS does not have Caller ID)
- does not call the police unless you ask them to
- is required by law to report suspected abuse, neglect, or dependency to DSS
- is not connected to any religious organization
- does not judge callers
- does not go out and look for kids
- gives messages to families
- will arrange conference calls between a minor and her family
- refers kids to shelter, food, and medical/legal assistance
- works with Greyhound Lines, Inc. to send kids home by bus through the Home Free program

Can I stay in school if I am homeless?

Whether you are homeless along with your parents or by yourself, there are special rules schools must follow to help you stay in school or get back to school. [Your rights as a homeless student are discussed in Chapter 59.]

✔ Quick Tip

The National Runaway Switchboard (NRS)—800-RUNAWAY, http://www.nrscrisisline.org—tries to help minors anywhere in the United States who have run away from home (or are thinking about it) or who are homeless for any reason.

Chapter 55

Second Chance Homes For Teen Mothers And Their Children

What are they?

Second Chance Homes are adult-supervised, supportive group homes or apartment clusters for teen mothers and their children who cannot live at home because of abuse, neglect, or other extenuating circumstances. Second Chance Homes can also offer support to help young families become self-sufficient and reduce the risk of repeat pregnancies. They provide a home where teen mothers can live, but they also offer program services to help put young mothers and their children on the path to a better future. Several federal resources are available to help state and local governments and community-based organizations create Second Chance Homes that provide safe, stable, nurturing environments for teen mothers and their children.

Second Chance Homes programs vary across the country, but generally include the following:

• an adult-supervised, supportive living arrangement

• pregnancy prevention services or referrals

About This Chapter: Information in this chapter is from "About Second Chance Homes," September 2001, U.S. Department of Housing and Urban Development.

- a requirement to finish high school or obtain a GED (general educational development)

- access to support services such as child care, health care, transportation, and counseling

- parenting and life skills classes

- education, job training, and employment services

- community involvement

- individual case management and mentoring

- culturally sensitive services

- services to ensure a smooth transition to independent living

Why are they important?

Second Chance Homes offer a nurturing home for society's most vulnerable families, teen mothers, and their children with nowhere else to go. Almost half of all poor children under six are born to adolescent parents. Children of teen mothers are 50 percent more likely to have low birth weight, 33 percent more likely to become teen mothers themselves, and 2.7 times more likely to be incarcerated than the sons of mothers who delay childbearing. Teen mothers are half as likely to earn their high school diplomas or GEDs and are more likely to be on welfare than mothers who are older when they give birth. In addition, research shows that over 60 percent of teen parents have experienced sexual and/or physical abuse, often by a household member. Limited early findings indicate that residents of Second Chance Homes have fewer repeat pregnancies, better high school/GED completion rates, stronger life skills, increased self-sufficiency, and healthier babies.

Second Chance Homes help teen mothers and their children comply with welfare reform requirements. Under the 1996 welfare law, an unmarried parent under 18 cannot receive welfare assistance unless she lives with a parent, guardian, or adult relative. However, if such a living arrangement is inappropriate (for example, if her family's whereabouts are unknown or if she was abused), states may waive the rule and either determine her current living arrangement to be appropriate, or help her find an alternative adult-supervised

✤ It's A Fact!!

Teen mothers can be referred to Second Chance Homes through welfare agencies, homeless shelters, foster care programs, or by community organizations, schools, clinics, or hospitals. Mothers may also self-refer.

supportive living arrangement such as a Second Chance Home. Also, in states where alternatives such as Second Chance Homes are currently not available, teen mothers could be forced to choose between inappropriate living arrangements and losing their cash assistance. Making Second Chance Homes available to teen mothers in need could provide these teens with stable housing, case management, and preparation for independent living.

Second Chance Homes can support teen families who are homeless or in foster care. State foster care systems may not have the capacity to place the teens and their children together, and frequently, homeless shelters, battered women's shelters, and transitional living facilities cannot accept teen parents under age 17. Unfortunately, homelessness poses the threat of separation in young families. For vulnerable families with no safe, stable places to go, Second Chance Homes can help fill the gap.

Who is eligible?

Eligibility criteria for Second Chance Homes vary from program to program. Some programs are targeted for adolescent mothers (between the ages of 14 to 20, for example), mothers receiving welfare assistance, or homeless families. Other programs are open to any mother in need of a place to live regardless of age, income, or the assistance program for which she qualifies.

Where are they?

Nationwide, at least six states have made a statewide commitment to Second Chance Home programs: Massachusetts, Nevada, New Mexico, Rhode Island, Texas, and Georgia. In statewide networks, community-based organizations operate the homes under contract to the states and deliver the services. States share in the cost of the program, refer teens to homes, and set standards and guidelines for services to teen families. In addition, there are many local Second Chance Home programs operating in an estimated 25 additional states.

What federal resources are available?

State legislatures may allocate Temporary Assistance to Needy Families (TANF) block grant funds for Second Chance Homes. Like TANF, state maintenance-of-effort (MOE) funds and the Social Services Block Grant (SSBG) are flexible and largely under states' discretion in terms of how they are spent. States and communities may also explore other sources of funding from the U.S. Department of Health and Human Services (HHS) and U.S. Department of Housing and Urban Development (HUD.) Additional state and private sources of funding are available to fill in funding gaps, help providers acquire or rehabilitate Second Chance Homes, or develop specialized Second Chance Homes for teen parents who are homeless or in foster care.

Where can I learn more?

A chart of major resources, both from the HHS and HUD, available to the program and funding information may be found at http://www.hud.gov/offices/pih/other/sch/resources.cfm. More general information on the program may be found at the Administration for Children and Families (http://www.acf.hhs.gov) and the Department of Housing and Urban Development (http://www.hud.gov).

Chapter 56

Child Custody

What is a custody order?

A custody order is a written order signed by a judge, determining who will care for a child and who gets to make important decisions about the child. There are two types of custody: physical and legal custody. The person awarded custody is called the custodian or custodial parent.

What are the advantages to having a custody order?

A custody order sets clear terms for when each parent can see and have the child with them. If one of the parents does not stick to the terms of the order, the other parent can file a petition with the court asking to find the other party in contempt and to enforce the order. The police or sheriff's office may also help enforce a custody order.

If no custody order exists, neither parent can keep the child away from the other parent. That means that if one parent takes the child out for the day and then will not return the child home, the police cannot force one parent to give the child to the other parent. A parent could only go down and file an emergency custody petition.

Parents who are having a hard time getting along and agreeing to things may benefit from getting a custody order.

About This Chapter: Information in this chapter is from "Young Parent's Custody Rights," © 2007 Juvenile Law Center. All rights reserved. Reprinted with permission.

What are the disadvantages to having a custody order?

When there is no custody order both parents basically have equal rights to the child and can, on there own, decide who the child is going to live with and when. When you have a custody order the court is involved in the life of your family. To change the terms of the order you may need to go back to court. Also, starting a custody action with the court sometimes gives the other parent an opportunity to get some custody or visitation when that parent has not been doing so on his or her own.

✎ What's It Mean?

Types Of Custody

Physical custody determines whom the child lives with. There are four types of physical custody:

1. **Primary:** The person who has the child living with them for most of the time

2. **Partial:** Gives the non-primary custodian the right to have the child live with them for parts of the week (weekends, for example) or year (vacations)

3. **Visitation:** Gives the non-custodial parent the right to go see the child, but not the right to take the child overnight. Visitations may be supervised by the custodial parent, a family member, or a responsible adult.

4. **Shared/Joint:** Gives shared legal or physical custody (or both) of the child

Legal custody gives the custodian the legal right to make important decisions such as medical, religious, and educational decisions.

Can a minor file for custody or initiate a custody proceeding?

All parents, including teen parents, have the right to seek custody or visitation of their children. In some states, however, a minor cannot file for custody on his or her own. To file for custody, a minor parent must file through an adult who is called a guardian.

Who can act as a guardian for filing custody?

The guardian must be over the age of 18, must accompany the minor party to all court proceedings, and must sign all court documents along with the minor parent. Even though the guardian files the custody petition, it is still the minor who is seeking custody.

The guardian does not have to be a caretaker to or have legal rights as a parent or guardian to the minor parent filing for custody. The guardian can be a family friend or social worker.

How do I prepare for a hearing?

To prepare for a hearing, you need to get ready to present testimony, evidence, and witnesses that help you show why the custody arrangement you are asking for is best for your child.

Testimony: Each party may present their side and ask questions of the other party. Each party should prepare and bring a list of their main points and any questions that they may have for the other party.

Evidence: This includes school, medical records, photographs, or other important documents. Each party has the right to see everything that the other side wants to show the court. Two copies of all documents should be made—the judge gets the original, and both parties get a copy.

Witnesses: Parties may bring witnesses to testify on their behalf. A witness must present a subpoena to be admitted into the court. Court employees can direct parties to where subpoenas can be obtained. Upon entering the courthouse, the witness must show it to the security guard. Each party should prepare a list of questions to ask their own witnesses and the witnesses of the other party. A letter from a witness is usually not enough; the person must actually come to the hearing.

What does the court consider in determining a custody order?

After a hearing is held, the judge decides the custody arrangement based on the Best Interests Standard—what is best for the child's physical, intellectual, and emotional well-being.

Things that the court MUST consider when making a custody decision are as follows:

- which parent will permit regular contact with the child and non-custodial parent
- each parent and household member's present or past abusive contact
- convictions of certain crimes
- the child's preference

Things that the court may consider when making a custody decision are as follows:

- who has been the child's primary caretaker and where the child is currently living
- the living environment of each party, including home, school, and the community
- where the child's siblings live
- drug and alcohol abuse or mental health issues
- work schedules of the parties

Chapter 57

If You Need Help Getting Child Support

The Child Support Enforcement (CSE) Program

The CSE Program is a government program to help make parents support their children when they do not live together. Federal, state, and local agencies work together to try to collect child support payments for you.

Who Can Use The CSE Program

Any father or mother who is the custodial parent or other adult who has custody of a minor and needs help with the following can use the program:

- locating where the noncustodial parent lives

- establishing whom the natural father is and how to prove it

- establishing the child support order or how much child support payment will be received

- enforcing the order or making sure child support payments are made

The CSE Program is also for the following:

About This Chapter: Information in this chapter is from *Giving Hope and Support to America's Children*, Administration for Children and Families, Office of Child Support Enforcement, U.S. Department of Health and Human Service (www.acf.dhhs.gov), 2000; cited November 2006.

- a father who needs help to establish paternity in order to have a legal relationship with a child

- a noncustodial parent who wants to establish a child support order or to pay child support through the CSE program

- a custodial parent who wants to collect payments after the child is 18

How Much Do CSE Services Cost?

If you are now receiving financial assistance through Temporary Assistance for Needy Families (TANF), Medicaid, or Federally-Assisted Foster Care Program, you qualify to receive free services from the CSE Program.

If you are not receiving financial assistance from any of these programs, you may have to pay a fee of no more than $25.00. Some states pay for part or all of the cost. Ask your caseworker or call your local child support office.

If you have the money, you may want to hire an attorney instead of using the services from the child support enforcement offices to collect child support payments.

How To Find The Noncustodial Parent

A noncustodial parent is a parent who does not live with a child. That person will usually be ordered to financially support the child. To start the process for child support, you must first find the noncustodial parent. In order to do this you will need a social security number, an address of current or recent employer, names of relatives, employers,

> **✔ Quick Tip**
>
> The following will help you during your request for child support:
>
> - full name of noncustodial parent (including other names or nicknames)
>
> - telephone number and complete address
>
> - social security number
>
> - date and place of birth
>
> - physical description
>
> - information about salary earnings or assets of the noncustodial parent such as pay slips, bank statements, property, or Form 1099
>
> - divorce papers or separation agreement

or friends who might know where the noncustodial parent lives, the birth certificate of the child, and a copy of the child support order or any previous order.

Where To Go To Receive More CSE Information

Call the CSE office in your state. In most states, the telephone call is free. If you do not find an office near you, check the county listings in your telephone book or write to the child support office in your state.

Once you have contacted the child support enforcement office near you, a person (caseworker) will be assigned to you.

If necessary, your caseworker will try to locate the parent through the Federal or State Parent Locator Service (FPLS or SPLS).

If the person lives in another state, through a new law called the Uniform Interstate Family Support Act (UIFSA), agencies in different states work together to enforce child support orders.

Once the noncustodial parent is found, the child support enforcement office will notify him that you want child support. The caseworker will ask the noncustodial parent to come for an interview or let this person know you plan to take legal action to get a child support order.

How To Establish Paternity

Establishing paternity is determining who is the natural father. Child support cannot be ordered without establishing paternity. It is important for children because they can obtain the following:

- a part of any social security retirement or disability benefits their father receives

- life insurance and inheritance their father might provide

- information about any health problems in their father's family

The best time to establish paternity is right after the child's birth, but it can be established at any time until the child is 18.

The father can sign an affidavit or a consent order saying that he is the father. If he will not do so, they can arrange to have the man take a blood or saliva test to determine if he is the father. The mother and the child will have to be tested also. These tests are called "genetic tests."

The following is a list of information and documents to help you establish paternity:

- letters or notes that might help prove who is the father
- pictures of the father with the children or the family
- proof of any money that the father has given to you or the child
- birth certificate signed by the father or some proof from the hospital that the father admitted paternity
- any birthday cards or Mother's Day cards that the father might have given to you or your child

In some states the father pays for genetic testing, and in others the mother pays if she is not receiving Temporary Assistance for Needy Families (TANF), Foster Care, or Medicaid.

Your caseworker can help file for a hearing to establish paternity if the father threatens to leave the state. If the father has been told of the hearing date according to state law, but does not appear, paternity can be established by default. A default judgment means that the law decides who is the father.

If you are concerned about the safety of your child, talk to your caseworker about how you can show that there is good cause for not giving the father's name; for example, the father has been violent with you or your child.

How To Establish A Child Support Order

The child support order may include benefits such as the amount of child support that must be paid, a medical insurance plan, additional medical costs not covered by insurance, provision for a child's support in case the parent dies, and financial support for an extended period of time for a child with disabilities.

✤ It's A Fact!!

Many states have agreements with foreign countries that recognize child support orders.

The following is a list of documents that will help you get a child support order:

• information such as paychecks, which show your own earnings and information about your assets (e.g., property, car)

• records of any money the noncustodial parent has given to you or your child

Each state has guidelines for determining child support payments. Many state guidelines consider special needs such as day care, special medical needs, and the amount of time a child spends with each parent.

Any parent can ask for a review of the child support order every three years, or if there is an increase or decrease of income, or change in a child's needs.

Your support order may be affected in some states if the noncustodial parent has another family. When there are two orders for support and the noncustodial parent's income is not high enough to pay both, the state should have a formula for sharing the available money between both orders.

If the noncustodial parent is in the military, your child should be included in their medical coverage.

How To Enforce The Order

When a parent is not helping to provide for his children, enforcement of the order becomes necessary. To enforce the child support order, you will need proof of the order.

The following are ways to enforce child support orders:

• If the parent has a regular job, money can be withheld from his paycheck whether or not he works in the same state you live in.

• If wage withholding does not work, and the parent is not paying, the CSE Program can take away the noncustodial parent's drivers, recreational, or occupational license.

- The CSE Program can take state and federal income tax refunds to repay past due support and can get liens on property and assets.

If the noncustodial parent is in jail, it is possible that he will not be able to pay child support; but if he is working from the jail and is earning money, you might be able to collect part of it. Once the noncustodial parent is released, he can start payments as soon as he starts working again.

If the noncustodial parent is in the military, the parent still needs to comply with wage withholding orders.

It is a federal crime if the noncustodial parent lives in another state and does not pay child support. If the parent owes more than $5,000, or has not paid for more than one year, ask your caseworker if the case can be forwarded to the U.S. Attorney's Office in your state.

Ask your caseworker for more information if the following is true:

- The noncustodial parent has his own business.

- The noncustodial parent's employer pays in cash.

- The noncustodial parent does not pay on time.

- The noncustodial parent tries to avoid paying by putting income or assets under a different name.

- Gifts in cash are given instead of payment.

- The noncustodial parent declares bankruptcy.

Chapter 58

Teen Fatherhood:
Rights And Responsibilities

There is a lot of advice out there for girls who find themselves facing an unwanted or unexpected pregnancy, but there is very little information out there for guys. It takes two to make a baby; but all too often when the pregnancy is announced, the guy gets lost in the confusion. Teen fatherhood is not something to be taken lightly, and along with responsibilities to the mother and the child, you have rights that you need to know about.

What are your rights as a prospective father?

First and foremost you have the right to know for sure that you are the father. This is not only a right you have, but it is a right that the unborn child is entitled to as well.

Understandably, a pregnant girl may be upset when the subject of DNA testing comes up, but it is not something you should ever feel guilty about requesting. You are not calling her sexual conduct into question by wanting to know for sure that you are the father. You are not suggesting that she is bad or a liar. You are simply exercising your right to know for sure that you are the father, and this is important because fatherhood is a lifelong commitment.

About This Chapter: Information in this chapter is from "Teen Fatherhood FAQ." © 2006 by Mike Hardcastle. Used with permission from About, Inc., which can be found online at www.about.com. All rights reserved.

If you are the father, you have the right to know your child and to participate in your child's life. You have rights of custody and access. You also have responsibilities. You have the responsibility to financially and emotionally care for your child. You have a responsibility to be present in your child's life and ensure that your child's needs are met. You have the responsibility to ensure that your child is safe and well cared for and is free from harm. You have the responsibility to make decisions that are in the best interest of your child. More on rights and responsibilities later; first lets look at the most important thing every prospective father needs to know about—how to know if they are really the father.

> **♣ It's A Fact!!**
> While everyone is mixed up in the emotionally charged circumstances surrounding an unwanted pregnancy, it is often overlooked or downplayed that both father and child have a right to know the truth about paternity.

How can you know if you are the father?

There are two ways to determine if you are the father, blood type matching and DNA testing. Blood type matching is the cheapest and simplest test, but it does not determine paternity. It only tells you if it is possible that you are the father. If the blood types do not match up, there is no possible way you are the father and no other tests are needed. If the blood types do match up, it only means that you could be the father, and a DNA test will be needed to know for sure.

In order to match blood types you need to know the answers to three questions: what is the father's blood type, what is the mother's blood type, and what is the baby's blood type? A baby's blood type is determined by the blood types of its parents, and it is an exact science as to what possible blood type a baby can have based on the types of the parents. It may sound confusing, but it is really very simple. The blood type of the baby is determined by a combination of its parents' blood types. If the baby has a blood type that could not be the result of the combined blood types of both parents, then the paternity is usually called into question (since in natural conception maternity is never at issue).

So what is the difference between a positive and a negative blood type match? Rh factor aside (which determines if the blood type is positive or negative and is not effected by paternity), a baby will have the same blood type as either its mother or its father or it will have a combined blood type based on the types of both parents. A negative blood type matching happens if a baby does not have the father's or mother's blood type or if the blood type that a baby does have is not a possible combination of the father's and the mother's. A positive blood type matching happens when a baby has the same blood type as the mother, the same blood type as the father, or a blood type that is a combination of the parent's blood types. Table 58.1 shows which blood types are possible based on the combined types of the parents.

Remember, in cases of natural conception, if the blood types do not match, it is because the wrong father has been identified. If the blood types do match up, the next step that should be taken is a DNA test, as blood type matches only suggest the possibility, not the certainty, that the right

Table 58.1. Determining Paternity By Blood Type

Parents' Blood Types	You May Be The Father If The Baby Is	You Are Not The Father If The Baby Is
A and A	A, O	B, AB
A and B	A, B, AB, O	All types match
A and AB	A, B, AB	O
A and O	A, O	B, AB
B and B	B, O	A, AB
B and AB	A, B, AB	O
B and O	B, O	A, AB
AB and AB	A, B, AB	O
AB and O	A, B	AB, O
O and O	O	A, B, AB

father has been identified. DNA testing is much more complicated and expensive, but in the end, it is worth the investment; and many private labs have payment programs available to make access to this test easier. Do not feel bad about wanting a DNA test; as discussed earlier, both father and a child have a right to know the truth. The most accurate DNA testing is done using samples from all three parties: mother, identified father, and child; but testing can be done with only samples from the identified father and child.

While it is possible to test DNA before a child is born, this is much more costly and can pose a risk to the unborn child. For this reason, most DNA testing is done after the child is born.

Should you get married?

The question of marriage under these circumstances is a very personal one, but it should not be entered into lightly. The pressure to marry when an unwanted pregnancy occurs can be overwhelming, but there are important legal ramifications that potential fathers must be aware of. In North America, our system of law is based on British Common Law; and under this legal structure, a child born in wedlock (that is to parents who are legally married at the time of birth) is automatically presumed to belong to the husband. A legal father has the same rights and responsibilities as a biological father. If you marry a girl who claims you fathered her child, and later find out that you are not the father, it can be difficult and costly, not to mention emotionally devastating, to have your parental rights and responsibilities changed. It may be worth your while to consult with a lawyer near where you live before marrying under these circumstances in order to fully and properly understand the law on this matter where you live.

What about adoption? Can I give up my baby for adoption even if the mother does not want to?

No. You cannot force the other parent to give the child up for adoption. You may be able to give up your own parental rights however, depending on the laws where you live. A lawyer in your area can better advise you on the subject of giving up parental rights and obligations; and if this is something you, want you must seek legal advice.

I'm the father, and I'm going to be involved, now what?

If you and the mother can agree on a custody arrangement and on child support, it can be as simple as signing an agreement and filing it with the family court in your area. This may or may not require a lawyer. When there is nothing being disputed by either parent, then the matter of filing is relatively simple, and any associated legal fees are usually minimal. If the two of you cannot agree, then you will need a lawyer. As a father you have the right to know your child and to be a participant in his or her life. You also have the responsibility to support and care for your child; and if you are the non-custodial parent, you have the responsibility to pay child support. As touched on earlier, you have the responsibility to ensure that your child is free from harm and is well cared for. If you believe that the mother is unable to care for your child or that your child is being harmed in her care, then you have a responsibility to do something about it. On the other hand, if a mother believes that you may be bad for the child or put the child in harms way, then she has a responsibility to do something about it. This usually involves going to court to stop or limit access. A lawyer will be needed, and depending on where you live, you may be able to get legal aid or assistance. Check with your local law society, Attorney General, or other public law office.

Parenthood is not an easy thing, and it should never be entered into lightly. No matter what the circumstances surrounding conception, when you become a parent, you are a parent for the rest of your life.

Just because biology has made it that mothers carry the child in their body, this does not mean that the mother is the most important parent. Both parents have important roles to play in the life of their child. While having a child while you are still a kid yourself is less than ideal, this does not make you any less a parent. Once you know a child is yours, it changes your life forever no matter how old, or young, you are.

☞ Remember!!
Fathers are no less important than mothers, and their obligations to their child are no less than those of a mother.

Chapter 59

Completing Your Education

Will I be able to stay in school while I am pregnant?

Yes. You have a right to stay in the same school, classes, and extracurricular activities you have been in or are eligible to enter. You do not have to change to a school or program that is for pregnant and parenting students. Your school cannot force you to change to another school or program, and it cannot make you uncomfortable enough to want to transfer or drop out. It would be illegal, for example, for school officials to tell you that they cannot make sure you will be safe in your current school now that you are pregnant.

If you do think you want to change schools or programs, consider asking the principal, teachers, and counselors at your current school whether the new program is as good as the one you are in now. You will want to know whether it offers the courses you need for college or a good job.

What if I have to miss school because of medical problems?

If your or your child's medical problem keeps you out of school, the school must excuse the absence. Be sure to ask the doctor to contact your school.

About This Chapter: Information in this chapter is from *Pregnancy and Parenting: A Legal Guide for Adolescents, Second Edition.* © 2006 University of North Carolina at Chapel Hill. Reprinted with permission. Note: "Staying in School" reflects federal and North Carolina law only. Most states have law on the points mentioned in the section and those laws vary. To see the document from which this excerpt was taken and three other legal guides on minors' pregnancy and parenting, go to http://www.teenpregnancy.unc.edu.

Although the absence will be excused, you will have to make up the work to get credit. If it is medically necessary for you to stay home for weeks or months, ask the school to arrange homebound instruction. You are legally entitled to it.

Why is it important to be in school as much as possible?

You will not learn as much from someone coming by your home briefly to teach you or bring you assignments, as you will from being in class. If you miss many school days, your grades may fall or you may lose credit, and you might even have to repeat a year.

If I am a parent, do I have rights at school?

Yes. First, you cannot be treated worse than other students for being a parent. For example, school boards cannot keep young parents out of extra-curricular activities. Second, schools must treat young mothers and fathers the same. So, fathers must be allowed to use school-related child care centers or take parenting classes too.

Can I drop out before age 16 because I'm pregnant or parenting or because my family needs me to work?

No. You must stay in school until you are 16. That is the law (although most lawyers think a married student can leave school at any age). Your parents are responsible for finding a way for you to attend school until age 16. You can ask the department of social services (DSS) for help in paying for child care and for information about licensed child care providers. If your parents cannot or will not help you arrange for child care so that you can go to school, call DSS, ask to speak to a Child Protective Services worker, and explain the problem.

Unless you are expelled, you have a legal right to stay in school until you are 21 years old or graduate, whichever comes first. So, even if you drop out for awhile, you can always return to school until you are 21.

If you do drop out, the school must tell you where else you could continue your education. That could be at an extended day program in the public school system, at the local community college, or somewhere else.

♣ It's A Fact!!

Pregnant and parenting teens that finish high school have higher rates of employment and higher pay. They are less likely to need government assistance, and their children are more likely to graduate from high school.

Can I go to school if I am homeless?

Yes. A federal law requires public schools to offer homeless students the same education as other students. The law applies whether you are homeless with or without your child and with or without your parent or guardian. These are the major things the law says:

- You are entitled to be in the regular school program, not just a program for homeless students. You are also entitled to any other school programs or services you need, including transportation to school and back; services for disadvantaged children, children with special needs, or students with limited English proficiency; vocational education; programs for gifted and talented students; and school meal programs.

- A school must let you in immediately even if you are by yourself and you do not have the records normally required for entering school (such as proof of residency, a birth certificate, your grades in the last school, or your immunization records).

- You have the right to help from the school district's liaison for homeless students. He or she can help you enroll, get transportation to and from school, and pursue other rights.

Can I finish high school at a community college?

Yes. But almost all community college students must be 16 years old. If you are 16, there are two ways to transfer:

1. If you have been out of school for several months (usually six months), you can enter community college if your parent, guardian, or legal custodian enrolls you.

2. You can transfer from school to community college any time after you are 16 if your school agrees that is best for you and the college lets you in. (This way does not require waiting for several months.) Ask the principal, a counselor, or someone else at school whether they can help you get these permissions.

Part Eight

If You Need Help Or More Information

Chapter 60

WIC: The Special Supplemental Nutrition Program For Women, Infants, And Children

What is WIC?

WIC provides nutritious foods, nutrition education, and referrals to health and other social services to participants at no charge. WIC serves low-income pregnant, postpartum, and breastfeeding women, infants, and children up to age five who are at nutrition risk.

WIC is not an entitlement program; that is, Congress does not set aside funds to allow every eligible individual to participate in the program. Instead, WIC is a federal grant program for which Congress authorizes a specific amount of funding each year for program operations. The Food and Nutrition Service, which administers the program at the federal level, provides these funds to WIC state agencies (state health departments or comparable agencies) to pay for WIC foods, nutrition education, and administrative costs.

Where is WIC available?

The program is available in all 50 states, 34 Indian tribal organizations, America Samoa, District of Columbia, Guam, Commonwealth Islands of

About This Chapter: Information in this chapter is from "WIC: The Special Supplemental Nutrition Program For Women, Infants, And Children," Food and Nutrition Service, U.S. Department of Agriculture, March 2006.

the Northern Marianas, Puerto Rico, and the Virgin Islands. These 90 WIC state agencies administer the program through 2,200 local agencies and 9,000 clinic sites.

Who is eligible?

Pregnant or postpartum women, infants, and children up to age five are eligible. They must meet income guidelines, a state residency requirement, and be individually determined to be at "nutrition risk" by a health professional.

To be eligible on the basis of income, applicants' income must fall at or below 185 percent of the U.S. Poverty Income Guidelines (currently $35,798 for a family of four). A person who participates, or has family members who participate in certain other benefit programs such as the Food Stamp Program, Medicaid, or Temporary Assistance for Needy Families (TANF), automatically meets the income eligibility requirement.

What is nutrition risk?

Two major types of nutrition risk are recognized for WIC eligibility. They are as follows:

- medically based risk such as anemia, underweight, overweight, history of pregnancy complications, or poor pregnancy outcomes

- dietary risks such as failure to meet the dietary guidelines or inappropriate nutrition practices

Nutrition risk is determined by a health professional such as a physician, nutritionist, or nurse and is based on federal guidelines. This health screening is free to program applicants.

How many people does WIC serve?

More than eight million people get WIC benefits each month. In 1974, the first year WIC was permanently authorized, 88,000 people participated. By 1980, participation was at 1.9 million; by 1985 it was 3.1 million; and by 1990 it was 4.5 million. Average monthly participation for Fiscal Year (FY) 2004 was approximately 7.9 million.

Children have always been the largest category of WIC participants. Of the 7.9 million people who received WIC benefits each month in FY 2004, approximately 4 million were children, 2 million were infants, and 1.9 million were women.

What food benefits do WIC participants receive?

In most WIC state agencies, WIC participants receive checks or vouchers to purchase specific foods each month that are designed to supplement their diets. A few WIC state agencies distribute the WIC foods through warehouses or deliver the foods to participants' homes. The foods provided are high in one or more of the following nutrients: protein, calcium, iron, and vitamins A and C. These are the nutrients frequently lacking in the diets of the program's target population. Different food packages are provided for different categories of participants.

Who gets first priority for participation?

WIC cannot serve all eligible people, so a system of priorities has been established for filling program openings. Once a local WIC agency has reached its maximum caseload, vacancies are filled in the order of the following priority levels:

- pregnant women, breastfeeding women, and infants determined to be at nutrition risk because of a nutrition-related medical condition
- infants up to six months of age whose mothers participated in WIC or could have participated and had a serious medical problem
- children at nutrition risk because of a nutrition-related medical problem
- pregnant or breastfeeding women and infants at nutrition risk because of an inadequate dietary pattern
- children at nutrition risk because of an inadequate dietary pattern
- non-breastfeeding, postpartum women with any nutrition risk
- individuals at nutrition risk only because they are homeless or migrants and current participants who, without WIC foods, could continue to have medical and/or dietary problems

What is the WIC infant formula rebate system?

Mothers participating in WIC are encouraged to breastfeed their infants if possible, but WIC state agencies provide infant formula for mothers who choose to use this feeding method. WIC state agencies are required by law to have competitively bid infant formula rebate contracts with infant formula manufacturers. This means WIC state agencies agree to provide one brand of infant formula, and in return, the manufacturer gives the state agency a rebate for each can of infant formula purchased by WIC participants. The brand of infant formula provided by WIC varies from state agency to state agency depending on which company has the rebate contract in a particular state.

♣ **It's A Fact!!**
WIC foods include iron-fortified infant formula and infant cereal, iron-fortified adult cereal, vitamin C–rich fruit or vegetable juice, eggs, milk, cheese, peanut butter, dried beans/peas, tuna fish, and carrots. Special therapeutic infant formulas and medical foods may be provided when prescribed by a physician for a specified medical condition.

By negotiating rebates with formula manufacturers, states are able to serve more people. For FY 2004, rebate savings were $1.64 billion, supporting an average of 2 million participants each month, or 25 percent of the estimated average monthly caseload.

Chapter 61

When You Need Help Paying For Child Care

Five Steps To Healthy Child Care Budgeting

Your child is priceless, but paying for good child care can be a struggle. In fact, child care is probably the second largest expense in your budget after rent or mortgage. Child care is expensive, but you may be able to reduce your child care costs or get some help paying your child care bills. Follow these steps to healthy child care budgeting.

Step One: Plan Ahead

Start thinking about child care options and costs as far in advance as possible—finding care or help with child care expenses can take some time.

Step Two: Call The Experts

This chapter will get you started, but a call to your local child care experts—your child care resource and referral (CCR&R) center—will give you a lot more information about child care financial assistance available in your community. Your CCR&R can also help you with finding and selecting child care and other parenting needs.

About This Chapter: Information in this chapter is from "Finding Help Paying for Child Care," 2003. Reprinted with permission from Child Care Aware, a program of NACCRRA. Childcareaware.org 1-800-424-2246.

Step Three: Be A Smart Consumer

Like all parents, you want the best for your child. You want your child to get the kind of care children need to be ready for school.

> ✔ **Quick Tip**
> Call 800-424-2246 or visit ChildCareAware.org to find the child care resource and referral (CCR&R) center in your area.

Child care is a big expense, so you want to make sure it is high quality. No matter what type of care you choose to buy—a child care center or care in someone else's home or your own home—use the "Check It Out" checklist in this chapter to help you evaluate it.

If you have good child care, the money you are paying is going for caregivers' salaries, so that they can stay in their jobs, and so that they can receive education and training that will help them best meet your child's care and early learning needs. Your child care fees are also helping to purchase food, toys, equipment, and supplies.

Once you have evaluated your child care setting or options, be an actively involved and informed consumer. Visiting and participating in events at your child's provider sends a strong message. It tells your child and your child's caregiver that you think what your child is doing and learning is important.

Step Four: Find Out What Kind Of Help May Be Available

Each type of child care financial assistance has different qualifications, like income level, employment status, or residency, so make sure you get all the facts. Some of the options are as follows:

- **State Child Care Subsidies:** Find out if you are eligible to receive state-funded child care subsidy. State child care subsidy is available in every state, but the eligibility guidelines vary. Usually, child care subsidies are available for lower-income families who are working, and in some cases, in school. If you are eligible, you pay part of the cost, and the rest is paid directly to your selected child care provider.

- **Local Programs:** Ask if your local government, United Way, or other community or faith-based organization provides child care scholarships.

- **Employer/College Support:** Does your employer (or college, if you are a student) provide child care scholarships, discounts to certain programs, or on-site child care at reduced rates?

- **Child Care Program Assistance:** Ask if your child care provider offers scholarships, discounts, or a sliding fee scale.

- **Pre-Kindergarten (Pre-K) Programs:** Many states now offer free or low cost pre-k programs for three and four year-old children. Eligibility requirements vary from state to state, but the goal of all pre-k programs is to make sure that children are better prepared for kindergarten. Pre-K programs are offered in public schools and other child care settings.

- **Head Start and Early Head Start:** Head Start and Early Head Start are federally, and sometimes state funded, full- or part-day programs that provide free child care and other services to help meet the health and school readiness needs of eligible children. Most, but not all, families who access Head Start or Early Head Start must have incomes that meet federal poverty guidelines.

- **Federal Earned Income Tax Credit (EITC):** You may be able to lower your taxes and even get up to several thousand dollars back if you qualify for the EITC. To qualify you must be working full- or part-time and make less than a certain amount based upon family size. You don't have to owe any taxes to get the EITC.

- **Federal Child Tax Credit (CTC):** If you have a dependent child under age 17, you may be able to get the Child Tax Credit, which can be worth hundreds of dollars per child. The income limit for the CTC is much higher than for the Earned Income Tax Credit, but you still don't have to owe any taxes to get the Child Tax Credit.

- **Federal Child and Dependent Care Tax Credit:** If you have a child under 13, and owe federal income taxes, this tax credit can help cover a portion or all of the taxes you owe if you qualify.

- **State Earned Income and Dependent Care Tax Credits:** Many states offer their own Earned Income or Child and Dependent Care tax credits. These credits are similar to the federal ones, except that in some states, you don't have to owe any taxes to get the State Child and Dependent Care credit. You can get both federal and state Earned Income and Child and Dependent Care credits.

- **Dependent Care Assistance Programs (DCAPs):** Your employer may offer a Dependent Care Assistance Program, which allows you to have money (up to $5,000 a year) taken out of your paycheck tax-free and put into a special account to be used for child care tuition reimbursement.

The main purpose of this type of program is to help you lower the amount of taxes you have to pay during the year. You should never put more money into this account than you will actually spend, because in most cases you will lose any leftover at the end of the year. You also can't claim any money you put in a DCAP for the Child and Dependent Care Tax Credit.

Step Five: Consider All Options

Think about what your family needs, and take a close look at your budget. Are there alternatives to paying for full-time child care? Is it possible or desirable to work fewer hours or share some hours of child care if you are in a two-parent household and working at different times? Could you share child care expenses with another family?

> **✔ Quick Tip**
> Visit ChildCareAware.org or call 800-424-2246 for more information on financial assistance and other child care and parenting resources.

The most important think is that your family and child are healthy and happy. By planning ahead, getting the facts, and using all of the resources available to help you—especially your local CCR&R—you are off to a good start in making the best choice for your family.

Check It Out!

Ask these questions to evaluate your child care options:

- Does the person who will be caring for your child have special training in early childhood education, first aid, and CPR (cardiopulmonary resuscitation)?

- How long has the caregiver been in the same program or providing child care in the home?

- Are just a few children being cared for by one caregiver (low child/adult ratio)?

- If there is more than one caregiver in the setting, is the total number of children in the group still fairly small (group size)?

- If you are considering a more formal child care program, is it nationally accredited, and is it state licensed or regulated?

- Does the caregiver welcome drop-in visits and parent ideas and involvement?

- Does the caregiver get on the children's eye level and give them lots of attention and encouragement?

- Are materials—such as books, blocks, toys, and art supplies—available to children all day long?

- Does the place look clean and safe, and is hand washing done often?

- Does the caregiver have written policies and procedures, including emergency plans?

- Does the caregiver have references?

- You know your child best—will your child be happy there?

✔ **Quick Tip**

An "Evaluating Child Care Worksheet" that has additional information and room for writing notes is available on the Child Care Aware Web site, ChildCareAware.org, or by calling 800-424-2246.

Chapter 62

Vaccines For Children Program

What is the history of the Vaccines for Children Program?

From 1989–1991, a measles epidemic in the United States resulted in tens of thousands of cases of measles and hundreds of deaths. Upon investigation, the Centers for Disease Control and Prevention (CDC) found that more than half of the children who had measles had not been immunized even though many of them had seen a health care provider.

In partial response to that epidemic, Congress passed the Omnibus Budget Reconciliation Act (OBRA) on August 10, 1993, creating the Vaccines for Children (VFC) Program. VFC became operational October 1, 1994. Known as section 1928 of the Social Security Act, the Vaccines for Children program is an entitlement program (a right granted by law) for eligible children age 18 and below.

VFC helps families of children who may not otherwise have access to vaccines by providing free vaccines to doctors who serve them.

VFC is administered at the national level by the CDC through the National Immunization Program. CDC contracts with vaccine manufacturers to buy vaccines at reduced rates.

About This Chapter: Information in this chapter is from "Parents and VFC," National Immunization Program, Centers for Disease Control and Prevention (CDC), May 2006.

States and eligible projects enroll physicians who serve eligible patients up to and including age 18 years and who provide routine immunizations with little to no out-of-pocket costs to the parents.

Which children are eligible?

Children who are eligible for VFC vaccines:

• are 18 years old or younger;

• are eligible for Medicaid;

• have no health insurance;

• are Native American or Alaskan Native; or

• they have health insurance, but it does not cover immunizations. (In these cases, these children must go to a Federally Qualified Health Center (FQHC) or Rural Health Clinic (RHC) for immunizations.)

Do I have to pay anything?

If your child meets one of the VFC eligibility criteria listed above, the vaccine must always be provided free of charge.

Free of charge means just that. The vaccines have already been paid for with federal tax dollars. This means that no one can charge a fee for the vaccine itself.

However, each state immunization provider has been granted (by law) the ability to charge what is called an "administrative fee." An administrative fee is similar to a patient's co-pay, in that it helps providers offset their costs of doing business.

The amount of the administrative fee differs from state to state based on a regional scale determined by the Centers for Medicare and Medicaid Services (CMS).

These regional administrative charges are maximum fees that providers may ask patients to pay. That means that if a state's administrative fee is $15.00, a provider may charge a patient any amount up to, but not exceeding that $15.00 charge, for each vaccine administered. There is no lower limit, so providers have the option to charge what they feel is fair, including no charge at all.

If a patient cannot afford to pay the administrative fee being charged by the provider, the law requires that the provider must still administer the vaccine to the patient. Parents of children enrolled in Medicaid programs should not be charged an administrative fee. To be reimbursed, the provider should bill the state Medicaid program.

What vaccines are provided?

The vaccines provided prevent the following diseases:

- diphtheria
- *Haemophilus influenzae* type b (Hib)
- hepatitis A
- hepatitis B
- influenza
- measles
- meningococcal disease
- mumps
- pertussis (whooping cough)
- pneumococcal disease
- polio
- rotavirus
- rubella (German measles)
- tetanus (lockjaw)
- varicella (chickenpox)

Where can I get these vaccines?

Your child can receive free vaccines provided through the VFC program at the following places:

- private doctors' offices
- private clinics

- hospitals

- public health clinics

- community health clinics

- some schools in some states

☛ **Remember!!**

The vaccines are totally free, but you may have to pay an administrative fee.

Chapter 63

Health Insurance Options For Women

What is health insurance and how does it affect me?

Health insurance is a formal agreement to provide and/or pay for medical care described in your health insurance policy. There are medical services that are not covered and will not be paid by your insurance company.

There are a variety of private and public health insurance programs. Most women obtain health insurance through their employer or as a dependent in a family plan. There also are public health insurance plans funded by the federal and state governments. However, there are 16 million uninsured women. As health insurance costs soar and employers cut benefits or jobs disappear, millions of people slip through the cracks and lose their coverage. These are working Americans who make too much money to qualify for Medicaid but do not have enough money to buy health insurance. Uninsured women are more likely to suffer serious health problems, partly because they tend to wait too long to seek treatment or preventive care. The lack of health insurance can even be deadly, as research has shown that uninsured adults are more likely to die earlier than those who have insurance.

About This Chapter: Information in this chapter is from "Health Insurance And Women," National Women's Health Information Center, U.S. Department of Health and Human Services, September 2004.

What are my health care options?

Private Health Insurance: People who have private insurance either buy it themselves or get it through their employer. Insurance obtained through an employer typically requires the employee to pay a small portion of the overall policy cost.

- **Fee-For-Service:** The provider gets paid for each covered service. Most have a deductible amount that you must pay each year before the insurance company will begin to pay for medical services.

- **Health Maintenance Organizations (HMOs):** They provide health services for a fixed monthly payment. The HMO Act of 1973 created this alternative to traditional health plans as a more affordable option.

- **Preferred Provider Organization (PPO):** This is another option that offers more choices than an HMO but can be more costly for out-of-network services.

Public Health Insurance: The government also provides health care coverage for qualifying women through Medicaid, Medicare, and special interest programs. These plans serve those who meet certain financial, age, or situational requirements. The following is a description of the different types of government health insurance programs:

- **Medicare:** This is the national health insurance program for people age 65 or older, some people under age 65 with certain disabilities, and people with permanent kidney failure. Medicare has two parts:

  - Part A covers inpatient hospital, skilled nursing, home health, and hospice services. Everyone over age 65 is entitled to Part A.

  - Part B covers outpatient hospital, physicians, lab, and other services. Part B is a supplemental policy that must be purchased.

  - The Medicare Modernization Act of 2003 provided for improved benefits and prescription drug coverage through low-cost plans. For more information, call 800-MEDICARE or go to http://www.medicare.gov.

- **Medicaid:** This is a state-run health program that receives federal funding and must meet federal guidelines regarding specific benefits. Medicaid provides health care to qualifying low-income individuals and families with limited resources. You must be a U.S. national, citizen, or permanent resident alien in order to apply for benefits. Each state defines its own eligibility rules and administers its own program services. Qualification in one state does not guarantee qualification in another state. For more information, call 877-267-2323 or go to http://www.cms.hhs.gov/medicaid.

Many states have become more flexible in their ability to serve families in need, especially if you fall into any of these categories:

- **Pregnant:** Both you and your child will be covered if you qualify.

- **Children/Teenagers:** May cover sick children or teenagers on their own.

- **Aged, Blind, and/or Disabled:** Nursing home and hospice care is available.

- **Leaving Welfare:** You may be eligible for temporary assistance.

- **State Children's Health Insurance Program (SCHIP):** This is a joint state and federal program that provides insurance for children of qualifying families. Families who make too much money to qualify for Medicaid but cannot afford private health insurance may be able to qualify for SCHIP assistance. Eligibility and health care coverage varies according to each state. For more information, contact http://www.insurekidsnow.gov or call 877-KIDS-NOW.

♣ It's A Fact!!

Families who make too much money to qualify for Medicaid but cannot afford private health insurance may be able to qualify for State Children's Health Insurance Program (SCHIP) assistance.

What if you are currently uninsured?

America's uninsured recently grew to more than 44 million people and most are in working families. To address to this problem, the government is looking for ways to provide more affordable health insurance and greater access to health care. Right now, there are a number of resources for women without health insurance. There are government-sponsored "safety net" facilities that provide medical services for those in need, regardless of ability to pay. "Safety net" facilities include community health centers, public hospitals, school-based centers, public housing primary care centers, and special needs facilities. The U.S. Department of Health and Human Services (HHS) recently awarded more than $19 million to expand and strengthen these facilities. For information on community health facilities, contact your local or state health department.

Other government-sponsored programs for uninsured women include the following:

- **Special Supplemental Nutrition Program for Women, Infants, and Children (WIC):** Provides supplemental foods, nutrition education, and referrals to health care for low-income pregnant, breastfeeding, and postpartum women, infants, and children up to age five. Contact: http://www.fns.usda.gov/wic.

- **Maternal and Child Health Bureau:** State programs provide health care services for low-income women who are pregnant and their children under age 22. The federal government funds these programs and establishes general guidelines regarding services. Each state determines eligibility and identifies the specific services to be provided. For services available in your area, contact http://mchb.hrsa.gov.

- **Indian Social Services Welfare Assistance:** Provides financial assistance for American Indians in need, living near or on reservations. Contact: http://www.doi.gov.

- **Projects for Assistance in Transition from Homelessness (PATH):** Federal grants are provided to states and territories that partner with local organizations to provide a variety of health services for homeless people who have serious mental illness. Contact: http://www.samhsa.gov.

Chapter 64

Directory Of Teen Pregnancy Resources

Information About Sexual Health, Pregnancy, And Birth

Advocates For Youth
2000 M Street NW, Suite 750
Washington, DC 20036
Phone: 202-419-3420
Fax: 202-419-1448
Website: http://
www.advocatesforyouth.org

American College of Nurse-Midwives
8403 Colesville Road, Suite 1550
Silver Spring, MD 20910
Phone: 240-485-1800
Fax: 240-485-1818
Website: http://www.midwife.org

American College of Obstetricians and Gynecologists (ACOG)
409 12th Street SW
P.O. Box 96920
Washington, DC 20024
Phone: 202-638-5577
Website: http://www.acog.org

American Pregnancy Association
1425 Greenway Drive, Suite 440
Irving, TX 75038
Toll Free: 800-672-2296
Fax: 972-550-0800
Website: http://
www.americanpregnancy.org
E-mail:
Questions@AmericanPregnancy.org

About This Chapter: Information in this chapter was compiled from many sources deemed reliable; inclusion does not constitute endorsement. All contact information was verified and updated in February 2007.

American Social Health Association

P.O. Box 13827
Research Triangle Park, NC 27709
Phone: 919-361-8400
Fax: 919-361-8425
Website: http://www.ashastd.org
Teen-oriented website: http://www.iwannaknow.org

Campaign for Our Children

1 N Charles, Suite 1100
Baltimore, MD 21201
Phone: 410-576-9015
Website: http://www.cfoc.org

Childbirth Connection

281 Park Avenue South, 5th Floor
New York, NY 10010
Phone: 212-777-5000
Fax: 212-777-9320
Website: http://www.childbirthconnection.org

Child Care Aware

3101 Wilson Boulevard, Suite 350
Arlington, VA 22201
Toll Free: 800-424-2246
Fax: 703-341-4101
TTY: 866-278-9428
Website: http://www.childcareaware.org

Child Welfare Information Gateway

Children's Bureau/ACYF
1250 Maryland Avenue, SW, Eighth Floor
Washington, DC 20024
Toll Free: 800-394-3366
Phone: 703-385-7565
Fax: 703-385-3206
Website: http://www.childwelfare.gov
E-mail: info@childwelfare.gov

Focus Adolescent Services

Toll Free: 877-362-8727
Phone: 410-341-4342
Website: http://www.focusas.com
E-mail: help@focusas.com

Alan Guttmacher Institute

120 Wall Street, 21st Floor
New York, NY 10005
Toll Free: 800-355-0244
Phone: 212-248-1111
Fax: 212-248-1951
Website: http://www.guttmacher.org
E-mail: info@guttmacher.org

Lamaze International

2025 M Street, Suite 800
Washington, DC 20036-3309
Toll Free: 800-368-4404
Phone: 202-367-1128
Fax: 202-367-2128
Website: http://www.lamaze.org
E-mail: info@lamaze.org

Life in the Fast Lane

http://www.teenageparent.org

March of Dimes

Pregnancy and Newborn Health
Service Center
1275 Mamaroneck Avenue
White Plains, NY 10605
Phone: (914) 997-4488
Website: http://
www.marchofdimes.com/pnhec/
pnhec.asp

National Black Women's Health Project

1420 K Street NW
Washington, DC 20005
Phone: 202-548-4000
Fax: 203-543-9743
Website: http://www.nbwhp.org
E-mail: nbwhp@nbwhp.org

National Campaign to Prevent Teen Pregnancy

1776 Massachusetts Avenue, NW,
Suite 200
Washington, DC 20036
Phone: 202-478-8500
Fax: 202-478-8588
Website: http://
www.teenpregnancy.org
E-mail:
campaign@teenpregnancy.org

National Institute of Child Health and Human Development (NICHD)

31 Center Drive
Bethesda, MD 20892-2425
Toll Free: 800-370-2943
Fax: 301-984-1473
TTY: 888-320-6942
Website: http://www.nichd.nih.gov

National Maternal and Child Health Clearinghouse

Parklawn Building
5600 Fishers Lane
Rockville, MD 20857
Toll Free: (888) 275-4772
Website: http://www.ask.hrsa.gov/
MCH.cfm
E-mail: ask@hrsa.gov

National Sexual Assault Hotline

Toll Free: 800-656-HOPE
(656-4673)

National Women's Health Information Center

8270 Willow Oaks Corporate Dr.
Fairfax, VA 22031
Phone: 800-994-9662
TDD: 888-220-5446
Website: http://
www.womenshealth.gov/Pregnancy

Providing Child Care For the Teen Parent

549 Bevier Hall
905 S. Goodwin Ave.
Urbana, IL 61801
Phone: 217-244-2849
Fax: 217-244-0191
Website: http://
www.urbanext.uiuc.edu/teencare

Sexuality Information and Education Council of the United States (SIECUS)

130 West 42nd Street, Suite 350
New York, NY 10036-7802
Phone: 212-819-9770
Fax: 212-819-9776
Website: http://www.siecus.org
E-mail: siecus@siecus.org

U.S. Department of Health and Human Services (HHS)

Administration for Children and Families
370 L'Enfant Promenade, SW
Washington, DC 20201
Website: http://www.acf.hhs.gov

Breastfeeding and Post-partum Support

International Lactation Consultant Association

1500 Sunday Dr.
Raleigh, NC 27607
Phone: 919-861-5577
Fax: 919-787-4916
Website: www.ilca.org
E-mail: ilca@erols.com

La Leche League International

1400 N. Meacham Rd.
P.O. Box 4079
Schaumburg, IL 60168-4079
Phone: 847-519-7730
Fax: 847-519-0035
Website: www.lalecheleague.org
E-mail: LLLHQ@llli.org

Nursing Mother's Counsel, Inc.

P.O. Box 50063
Palo Alto, CA 94303
Phone: 650-327-6455
Website: www.nursingmothers.org

Postpartum Education for Parents

P.O. Box 6154
Santa Barbara, CA 93160
Phone: 805-564-3888
Website: www.sbpep.org

Chapter 65

Directory Of Assistance Resources For Low-Income Pregnant Women

American Public Human Services Association
810 First Street NE, Suite 500
Washington, DC 20002
Phone: 202-682-0100
Fax: 202-289-6555
Website: http://www.aphsa.org

Centers for Medicare and Medicaid Services
7500 Security Boulevard
Baltimore, MD 21244-1850
Toll-Free: 877-267-2323
Toll Free TTY: 866-226-1819
Phone: 410-786-3000
TTY: 410-786-0727
Website: http://cms.hhs.gov

Free Medicine Foundation
P.O. Box 125
Doniphan, MO 63935-0515
Phone: 573-996-73007
Website: http://
www.freemedicinefoundation.com
E-mail: help@Freemedicine.com

National Academy for State Health Policy
50 Monument Square, Suite 502
Portland, ME 04101
Phone: 207-874-6524
Fax: 207-874-6527
Website: http://www.nashp.org
E-mail: info@nashp.org

National Advocates for Pregnant Women
39 West 19th Street, Suite 602
New York, NY 10011
Phone: 212-255-9252
Fax: 212-255-9253
Website: http://
advocatesforpregnantwomen.org
E-mail:
info@advocatesforpregnantwomen.org

National Association of Public Hospitals and Health Systems
1301 Pennsylvania Avenue NW
Washington, DC 20004
Phone: 202-585-0100
Fax: 202-585-0101
Website: http://www.naph.org
E-mail: naph@naph.org

National Coalition on Health Care
1200 G Street NW, Suite 750
Washington, DC 20005
Phone: 202-638-7151
Website: http://www.nchc.org
E-mail: info@nchc.org

National Rural Health Association
521 East 63rd Street
Kansas City, MO 64110
Phone: 816-756-3140
Website: http://www.nrharural.org
E-mail: mail@nrharural.org

Office of Rural Health Policy
5600 Fishers Lane, 9A55
Rockville, MD 20857
Phone: 301-443-0835
Fax: 301-443-2803
Website: http://
www.ruralhealth.hrsa.gov

Robert Wood Johnson Foundation
P.O. Box 2316
Princeton, NJ 08543
Phone: 888-631-9989
Website: http://www.rwjf.org

State Coverage Initiatives
1801 K Street NW, Suite 701-L
Washington, DC 20006
Phone: 202-292-6700
Fax: 202-292-6800
Website: http://
www.statecoverage.net
E-mail: info@academyhealth.org

Women, Infants, and Children (WIC)
3101 Park Center Drive, Room 520
Alexandria, VA 22302
Phone: 703-305-2746
Website: http://www.fns.usda.gov/
wic
Directory of Regional WIC
Offices: http://www.fns.usda.gov/
wic/Contacts/fnsoffices.htm
E-mail: wichq-web@fns.usda.gov

Chapter 66

Directory Of Education Resources For Teen Parents

National Resources

American Council on Education
One Dupont Circle, NW
Washington, DC 20036
Phone: 202-939-9300
Website: http://www.acenet.edu
GED Testing Service: http://
www.acenet.edu/AM/
Template.cfm?Section=GEDTS
E-mail: comments@ace.nche.edu

Job Corps
U.S. Department of Labor
Website: http://jobcorps.dol.gov

U.S. Department of Education
400 Maryland Avenue, SW
Washington, DC 20202
Toll Free: 800-872-5327
Fax: 202-401-0689
TTY: 800-437-0833
Websites: http://www.ed.gov

About This Chapter: Information in this chapter was compiled from many sources deemed reliable; inclusion does not constitute endorsement. All contact information was verified and updated in February 2007.

Online Directories For State-Specific Help

American Association of Community Colleges

Assists you in locating a community college that can serve your continuing education needs.

Website: http://www.aacc.nche.edu/Template.cfm?Section=Community CollegeFinder1

State Coordinator Of Education For Homeless Children And Youth

Ensures that all homeless children and youth have equal access to the same free, appropriate public education, including public preschool education, provided to other children and youth; develops, reviews, and revises policies to remove barriers to the enrollment, attendance, and success in school of homeless children and youth; provides them with opportunities to meet the same challenging state content and state student performance standards to which all students are held.

Website: http://wdcrobcolp01.ed.gov/Programs/EROD/org_list.cfm ?category_cd=SHC

State Director Of Adult Education

Provides students with opportunities to develop skills needed to qualify for further education, job training, and better employment.

Website: http://wdcrobcolp01.ed.gov/Programs/EROD/ org_list.cfm?category_cd=DAE

State Tech Prep Coordinator

Prepares students for a highly skilled, technical occupation that allows either direct entry into the workplace as a qualified technician or further education leading to baccalaureate and advanced degrees. Tech Prep is a four-year sequence of study from the 11th grade through two years of post secondary occupation education culminating in a certificate or associate degree.

Website: http://wdcrobcolp01.ed.gov/Programs/EROD/ org_list.cfm?category_ID=TPC

Financial Aid Information For Post-Secondary Education

Broke Scholar
100 City Hall Plaza, Level 3
Boston, MA 02108
Phone: 617-399-8000 x237
Fax: 617-399-8050
Website: http://
www.brokescholar.com

College Board Scholarship Search
45 Columbus Avenue
New York, NY 10023
Website: http://
apps.collegeboard.com/cbsearch_ss/
welcome.jsp

FastWeb
Website: http://www.fastweb.com

Federal Student Aid
Phone: 800-433-3243
TTY: 800-730-8913
Website: http://studentaid.ed.gov

FinAid
Website: http://www.finaid.org

Free Application for Federal Student Aid (FAFSA)
Phone: 800-4-FED-AID
(800-433-3243)
Phone: 319-337-5665
TTY: 800-730-8913
Website: http://www.fafsa.ed.gov

National Association of Student Financial Aid Administrators
Website: http://www.nasfaa.org

SallieMae
P.O. Box 9500
Wilkes-Barre, PA 18773-9500
Phone: (888) 2-SALLIE
(888-272-5543)
TDD: (888) TDD-SLMA
(888-833-7562)
Website: http://www.salliemae.com

Additional Reading About Education For Teen Parents

Career Education for Teen Parents
Eric Digest
URL: http://www.ericdigests.org/1995-2/teen.htm

Civil Rights of Pregnant and Parenting Teens in California Schools
California Women's Law Center
URL: http://www.cwlc.org/files/docs/policy_brief_civil_rights_ppt.pdf

Guidance on the Education of School Age Parents
Department for Educational Skills (UK)
URL: http://www.dfes.gov.uk/schoolageparents

Helping the Education System Work for Teen Parents and Their Children
Center for Assessment and Policy Development
URL: http://www.capd.org/pubfiles/pub-1999-10-06.pdf

Rights of Pregnant and Parenting Teens
New York Civil Liberties Union
URL: http://www.nyclu.org/rrp_rppt2.html

School-Based and School-Linked Programs for Pregnant and Parenting Teens and Their Children
U.S. Department of Education
URL: http://www.ed.gov/PDFDocs/teenparent.pdf

Schools Failing To Accommodate Teens Who Are Pregnant Or New Mothers
University of Illinois at Urbana-Champaign
URL: http://www.news.uiuc.edu/NEWS/04/0423pregnant.html

Index

Index

Page numbers that appear in *Italics* refer to illustrations. Page numbers that have a small 'n' after the page number refer to information shown as Notes at the beginning of each chapter. Page numbers that appear in **Bold** refer to information contained in boxes on that page (except Notes information at the beginning of each chapter).